# AIR FRYER
## COOKBOOK

Amazing recipes without the guilt

Publications International, Ltd.

**Pictured on the front cover**: Buttermilk Air-Fried Chicken *(page 70),* Kale Chips *(page 158),* and Sweet Potato Fries *(page 116).*

**Pictured on the back cover** *(clockwise from top left)*: Teriyaki Salmon *(page 60),* Veggie Pizza Pitas *(page 148),* Double-Berry Shortcakes *(page 184),* and Green Bean Fries *(page 104).*

ISBN: 978-1-64030-135-1

Manufactured in China.

8 7 6 5 4 3 2 1

**Microwave Cooking:** Microwave ovens vary in wattage. Use the cooking times as guidelines and check for doneness before adding more time.

# Table of Contents

# Enjoy your Air Fryer

Do you love fried foods but try to avoid them? You no longer need to worry.

The air fryer is your answer to preparing fried foods without the extra calories, fat, or mess in the kitchen. You'll get the taste, and texture of fried foods—crispy, tasty, and crunchy—that you love and crave, without the added guilt often felt when consuming them. Plus, you'll soon see how your air fryer is so easy to use, cooks food faster, and provides a no-fuss clean up.

You'll love the ability to prepare fried foods in your air fryer, but you'll also soon find that you can prepare all types of other foods, too. Make everything from appetizers to meals to sides and even desserts! Why not try cookies or muffins? What about trying marinated salmon or a tuna melt? You'll even love the taste of roasted vegetables. You can bake in it, grill in it, steam in it, roast in it, and reheat in it.

Choose from more than 80 ideas here, or create your own.

Now get started and have fun eating and serving all those healthier foods without the added guilt.

## Helpful Tips:

- Read your air fryer's manufacturer's directions carefully before cooking to make sure you understand the specific features of your air fryer before starting to cook.

- Preheat your air fryer for 2 to 3 minutes before cooking.

- You can cook foods typically cooked in the oven in your air fryer. But because the air fryer is more condensed than a regular oven, it is recommended that recipes cut 25°F to 50°F off temperature and 20% off the typical cooking times.

- Avoid having foods stick to your air fryer basket by using nonstick cooking spray or cooking on parchment paper or foil. You can also get food to brown and crisp more easily by spraying occasionally with nonstick cooking spray during the cooking process.

- Don't overfill your basket. Each air fryer differs in its basket size. Cook foods in batches as needed.

- Use toothpicks to hold food in place. You may notice that light foods may blow around from the pressure of the fan. Just be sure to secure foods in the basket to prevent this.

- Check foods while cooking by opening the air fryer basket. This will not disturb cooking times. Once you return the basket, the cooking resumes.

- Experiment with cooking times of various foods. Test foods for doneness before consuming—check meats and poultry with a meat thermometer, and use a toothpick to test muffins and cupcakes.

- Use your air fryer to cook frozen foods, too! Frozen French fries, fish sticks, chicken nuggets, individual pizzas—these all work great. Just remember to reduce cooking temperatures and times.

# Estimated Cooking Temperatures/Times*

| FOOD | TEMPERATURE | TIMING |
|---|---|---|
| Vegetables (asparagus, broccoli, corn-on-cob, green beans, mushrooms, cherry tomatoes) | 390°F | 5 to 6 min. |
| Vegetables (bell peppers, cauliflower, eggplant, onions, potatoes, zucchini) | 390°F | 8 to 12 min. |
| Chicken (bone-in) | 370°F | 20 to 25 min. |
| Chicken (boneless) | 370°F | 12 to 15 min. |
| Beef (ground beef) | 370°F | 15 to 17 min. |
| Beef (steaks, roasts) | 390°F | 10 to 15 min. |
| Pork | 370°F | 12 to 15 min. |
| Fish | 390°F | 10 to 12 min. |
| Frozen Foods | 390°F | 10 to 15 min. |

*This is just a guide. All food varies in size, weight, and texture. Be sure to test your food for preferred doneness before consuming it. Also, some foods will need to be shaken or flipped to help distribute ingredients for proper cooking.*

Make note of the temperatures and times that work best for you for continued success of your air fryer.

Enjoy and have fun!

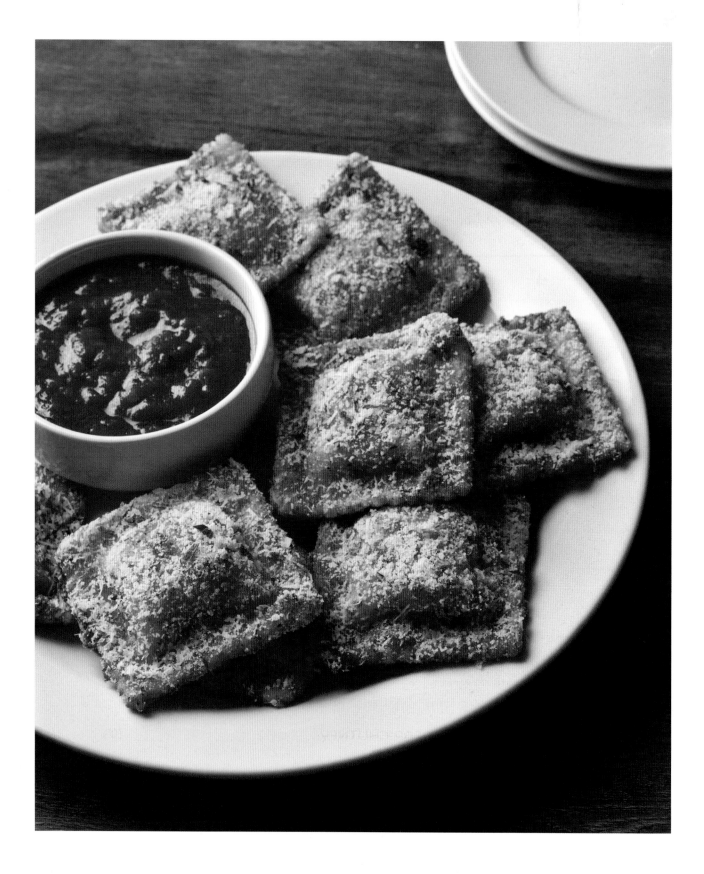

# Appetizers & Starters

# Fried Tofu with Sesame Dipping Sauce

3 tablespoons soy sauce or tamari

2 tablespoons unseasoned rice vinegar

2 teaspoons sugar

1 teaspoon sesame seeds, toasted*

1 teaspoon dark sesame oil

⅛ teaspoon red pepper flakes

1 package (about 14 ounces) extra firm tofu

¼ cup all-purpose flour

1 egg

1 cup panko bread crumbs**

Salt

*To toast sesame seeds, spread seeds in small skillet. Shake skillet over medium-low heat about 3 minutes or until seeds begin to pop and turn golden.

**Panko bread crumbs are used in Japanese cooking to provide a crisp exterior to foods. They are coarser than ordinary bread crumbs. Panko can be found in Asian markets or in the Asian aisle of supermarkets.

1. Whisk soy sauce, vinegar, sugar, sesame seeds, sesame oil and red pepper flakes in small bowl until well blended; set aside.

2. Drain tofu and press between paper towels to remove excess water. Cut crosswise into four slices; cut each slice diagonally into triangles. Place flour in shallow dish. Beat egg in shallow bowl. Place panko in another shallow bowl.

3. Dip each piece of tofu in flour, turning to lightly coat all sides. Dip in egg, letting excess drip back into bowl. Roll in panko to coat. Season with salt.

4. Preheat air fryer to 390°F. Spray tofu with nonstick cooking spray. Cook in batches 5 to 6 minutes or until golden brown. Serve with sauce for dipping.

MAKES 4 SERVINGS

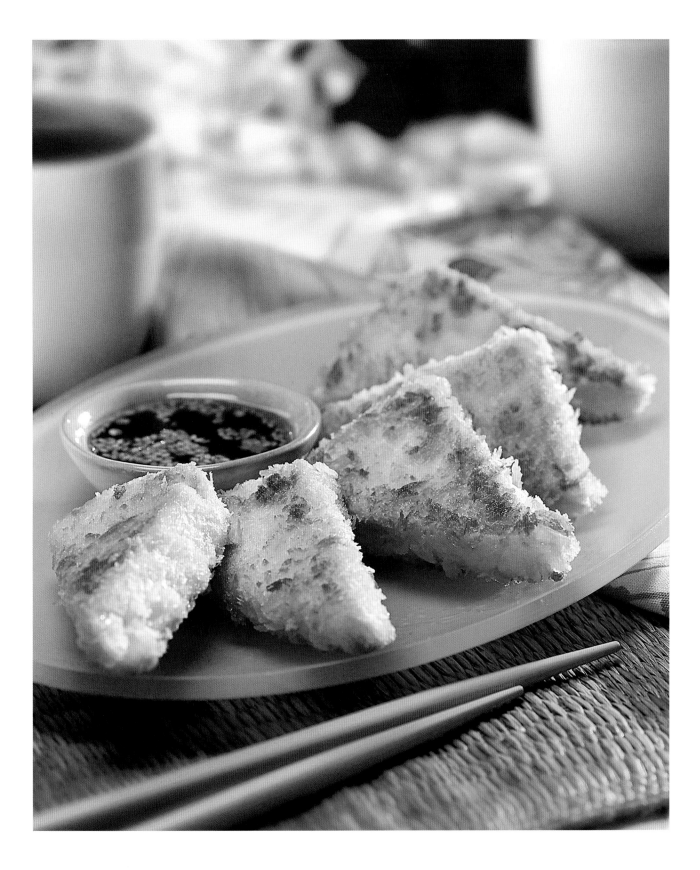

# Shanghai Chicken Wings

## SAUCE

½ cup water

½ tablespoon cornstarch

2 tablespoons packed dark brown sugar

2 tablespoons soy sauce

1½ tablespoons lime juice

1 tablespoon minced fresh ginger

½ teaspoon minced garlic

⅛ teaspoon red pepper flakes

## CHICKEN

1 cup all-purpose flour

¼ cup cornstarch

2 teaspoons salt

¼ teaspoon black pepper

¼ teaspoon ground red pepper

¼ teaspoon paprika

2 eggs

½ cup milk

1 pound chicken drummettes or wings

1. For sauce, whisk water and cornstarch in medium saucepan until smooth. Add brown sugar, soy sauce, lime juice, ginger, garlic and red pepper flakes; whisk until well blended. Bring to a boil over high heat. Reduce heat to low; simmer 10 minutes or until thickened, stirring occasionally. Transfer to large bowl; set aside to cool.

2. For chicken, combine flour, cornstarch, salt, black pepper, ground red pepper and paprika in large bowl. Whisk eggs and milk in shallow bowl. Coat chicken with flour mixture. Dip in egg mixture, letting excess drip back into bowl. Coat again with flour mixture. Spray chicken with nonstick cooking spray.

3. Preheat air fryer to 370°F. Cook in batches 16 to 18 minutes or until golden brown and cooked throughout, shaking halfway through cooking. Brush sauce over warm chicken. Remove to serving plate.

*MAKES 4 TO 6 SERVINGS*

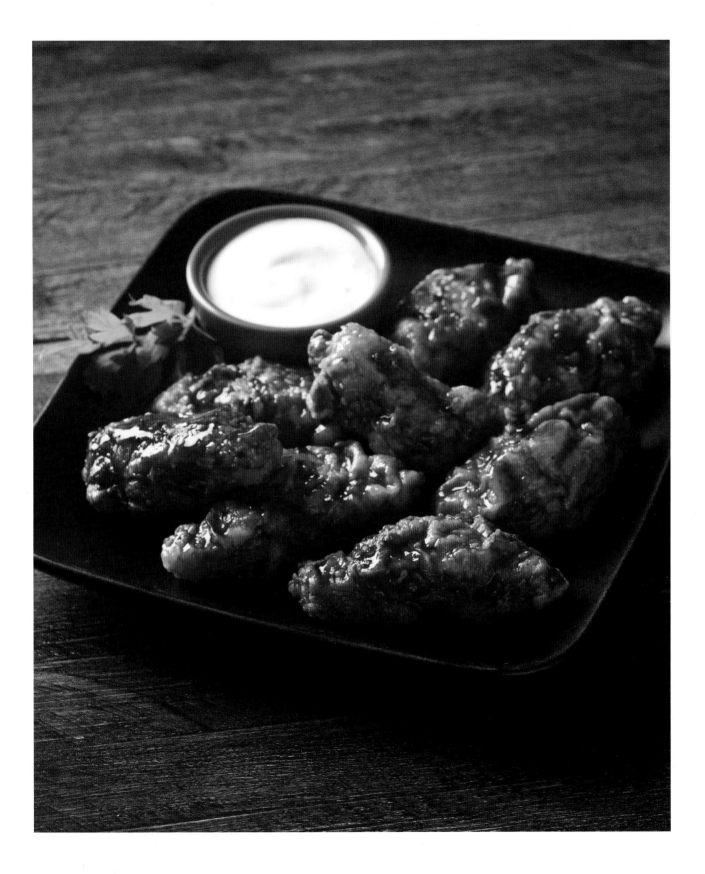

# Mozzarella Sticks

¼ cup all-purpose flour

2 eggs

1 tablespoon water

1 cup plain dry bread crumbs

2 teaspoons Italian seasoning

½ teaspoon salt

½ teaspoon garlic powder

1 package (12 ounces) string cheese (12 sticks)

1 cup marinara or pizza sauce, heated

1. Place flour in shallow bowl. Whisk eggs and water in another shallow bowl. Combine bread crumbs, Italian seasoning, salt and garlic powder in third shallow bowl.

2. Coat each piece of cheese with flour. Dip in egg mixture, letting excess drip back into bowl. Roll in bread crumb mixture to coat. Dip again in egg mixture and roll again in bread crumb mixture. Refrigerate until ready to cook.

3. Preheat air fryer to 370°F. Line air fryer with parchment paper; spray with nonstick cooking spray. Cook in batches 8 to 10 minutes or until golden brown, shaking halfway through cooking.

4. Serve with marinara sauce for dipping.

*MAKES 4 TO 6 SERVINGS*

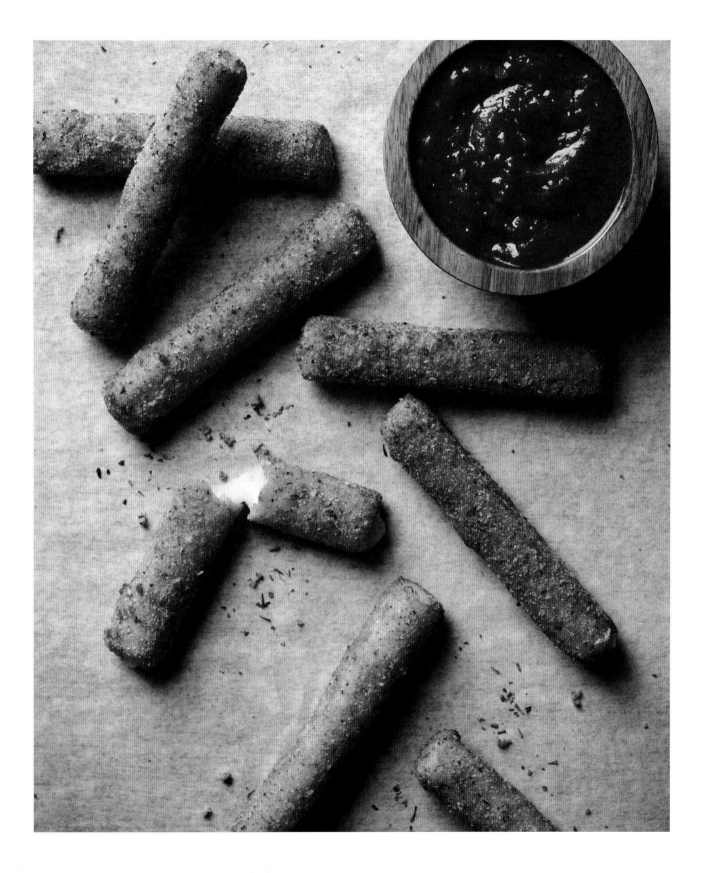

# Baked Orange Brie Appetizer

1 sheet frozen puff pastry (half of 17¼-ounce package)

⅓ cup orange marmalade

2 tablespoons chopped pecans (optional)

1 round (8 ounces) Brie cheese

1 egg white

1. Unfold puff pastry; thaw 20 minutes on lightly floured surface.

2. Preheat air fryer to 360°F.

3. Roll out puff pastry to 12-inch square. Use knife to cut off the four corners; set aside scraps.

4. Spread marmalade over center of pastry to 1 inch of edges. Sprinkle pecans over marmalade, if desired. Place Brie in center on top of pecans. Brush exposed dough with egg white.

5. Gather up edges of puff pastry and bring together over center of Brie, covering cheese entirely. Pinch and twist pastry edges together to seal. Use dough scraps to decorate top of Brie. Brush lightly with egg white. Transfer to air fryer basket.

6. Cook 8 to 10 minutes or until golden brown. (If top of pastry browns too quickly, cover loosely with small piece of foil.) Serve warm.

*MAKES 6 SERVINGS*

Variation: For added flavor and texture, sprinkle 2 tablespoons sliced almonds over the marmalade. Proceed with wrapping and cooking the Brie as directed.

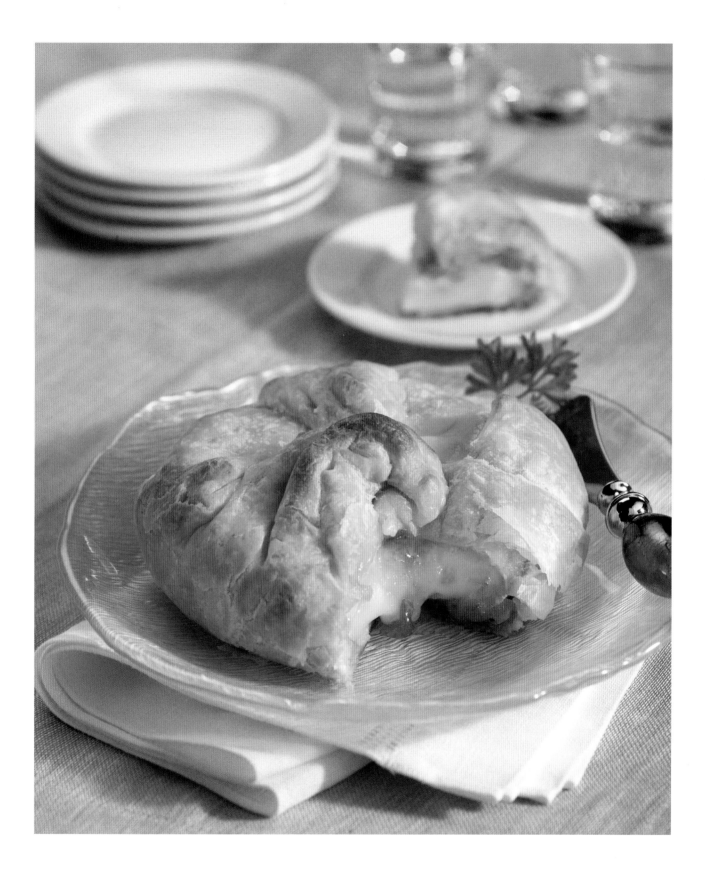

# Bacon-Wrapped Teriyaki Shrimp

1 pound large raw shrimp, peeled and deveined (with tails on)

¼ cup teriyaki marinade

11 to 12 slices bacon, cut in half crosswise

1. Place shrimp in large resealable food storage bag. Add teriyaki marinade; seal bag and turn to coat. Marinate in refrigerator 15 to 20 minutes.

2. Remove shrimp from bag; reserve marinade. Wrap each shrimp with 1 piece bacon. Brush bacon with some of reserved marinade.

3. Preheat air fryer to 400°F. Line air fryer basket with parchment paper or foil; spray lightly with nonstick cooking spray.

4. Cook 4 to 6 minutes or until bacon is crisp and shrimp are pink and opaque.

*MAKES 4 TO 5 SERVINGS*

Tip: Do not use thick-cut bacon for this recipe, because the bacon will not be completely cooked when the shrimp are cooked through.

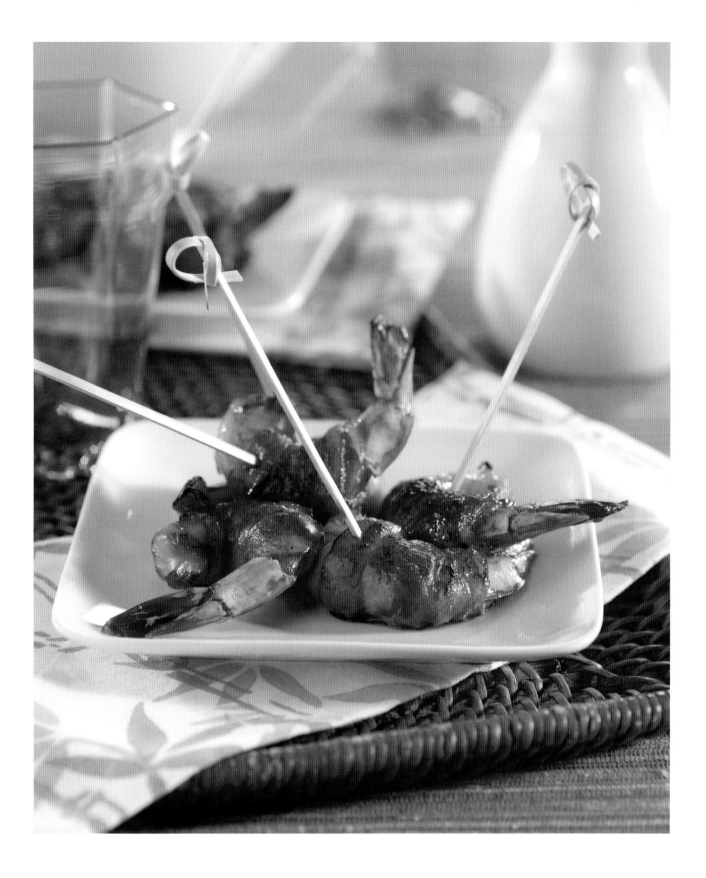

# Toasted Ravioli

1 cup all-purpose flour

2 eggs

¼ cup water

1 cup plain dry bread crumbs

1 teaspoon Italian seasoning

¾ teaspoon garlic powder

¼ teaspoon salt

½ cup grated Parmesan cheese

2 tablespoons finely chopped fresh parsley (optional)

1 package (10 ounces) meat or cheese ravioli, thawed if frozen

Pasta sauce, heated

1. Place flour in shallow bowl. Whisk eggs and water in another shallow bowl. Combine bread crumbs, Italian seasoning, garlic powder and salt in third shallow bowl. Combine cheese and parsley, if desired, in large bowl.

2. Preheat air fryer to 390°F. Poke holes in ravioli with toothpick.

3. Coat ravioli with flour. Dip in egg mixture, letting excess drip back into bowl. Roll in bread crumb mixture to coat. Spray with nonstick cooking spray.

4. Cook in batches 5 to 6 minutes or until golden brown, turning once. Add to bowl with cheese; toss to coat. Serve warm with sauce.

*MAKES 4 TO 5 SERVINGS*

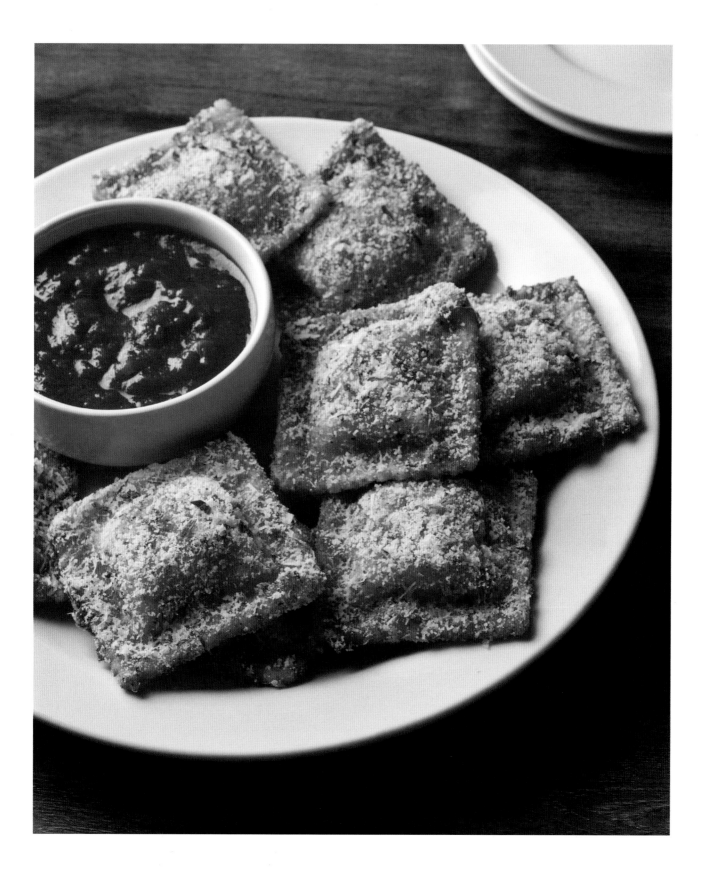

# Plum-Ginger Bruschetta

1 sheet frozen puff pastry (half of 17¼-ounce package)

2 cups chopped unpeeled firm ripe plums (about 3 medium)

2 tablespoons sugar

2 tablespoons chopped candied ginger

1 tablespoon all-purpose flour

2 teaspoons lemon juice

⅛ teaspoon ground cinnamon

2 tablespoons apple jelly or apricot preserves

1. Unfold puff pastry; thaw 20 minutes on lightly floured surface.

2. Preheat air fryer to 360°F. Line air fryer basket with parchment paper.

3. Cut puff pastry sheet lengthwise into 3 strips. Cut each strip crosswise in thirds to make 9 pieces. Cook in batches 5 to 6 minutes or until puffed and lightly browned.

4. Meanwhile, combine plums, sugar, ginger, flour, lemon juice and cinnamon in medium bowl.

5. Gently brush each puff pastry piece with about ½ teaspoon jelly; top with scant ¼ cup plum mixture. Cook in batches 1 to 2 minutes or until fruit is tender.

*MAKES 9 SERVINGS*

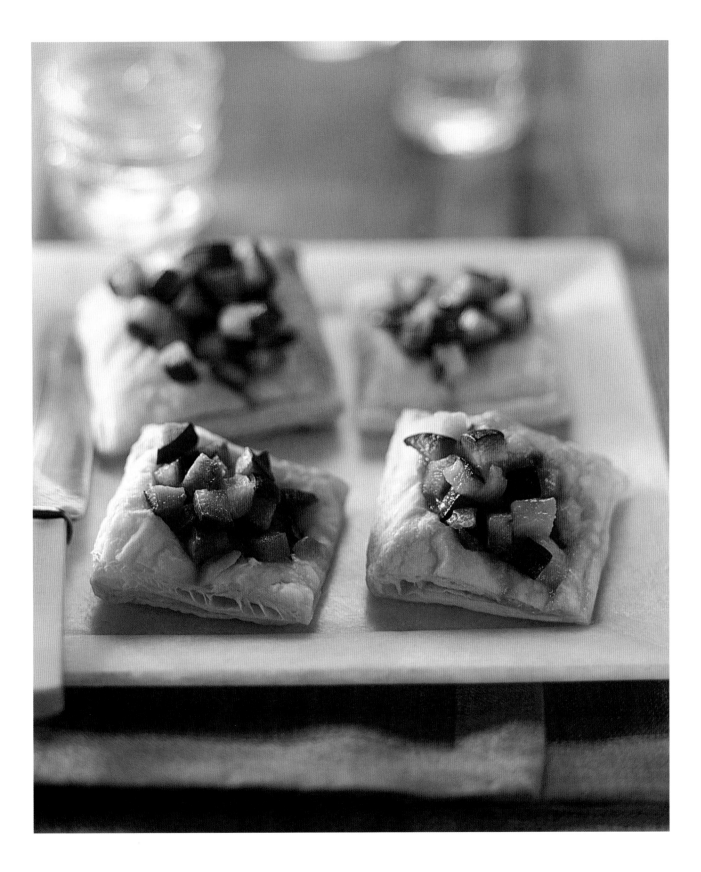

# Caprese-Style Tartlets

3 tomatoes, cut into 4 slices each

3 tablespoons pesto sauce

1 sheet frozen puff pastry (half of 17¼-ounce package)

6 ounces fresh mozzarella cheese

2 tablespoons chopped kalamata olives

1. Place tomatoes in large resealable food storage bag. Add pesto; toss to coat. Marinate at room temperature 30 minutes.

2. Unfold puff pasty; thaw 20 minutes on lightly floured surface.

3. Preheat air fryer to 350°F. Line air fryer basket with parchment paper.

4. Cut out six 4-inch rounds from pastry. Top each round with two tomato slices. Cook in batches 7 to 8 minutes or until pastry is light golden and puffed.

5. Cut mozzarella into six ¼-inch-thick slices. Top each tart with one mozzarella slice. Cook in batches 1 minute or until cheese is melted. Top tarts evenly with olives. Serve warm.

*MAKES 6 TARTLETS*

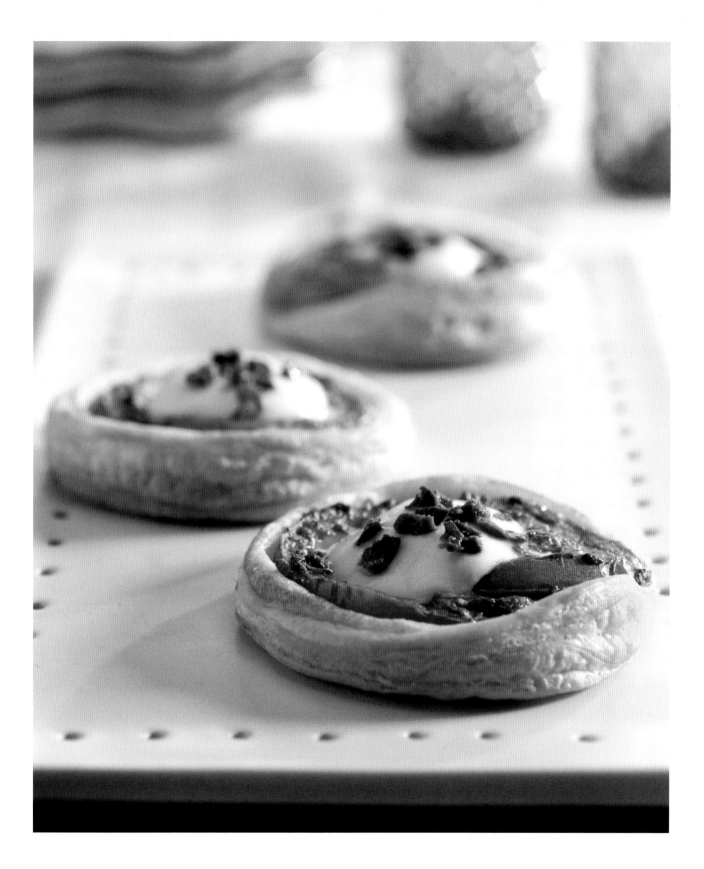

# Spinach Cheese Bundles

1 package (17¼ ounces)
    frozen puff pastry
    (2 sheets)

1 package (6½ ounces)
    garlic-and-herb
    spreadable cheese

½ cup packed chopped
    spinach

¼ teaspoon black pepper

    Sweet and sour sauce
    (optional)

1. Unfold puff pastry; thaw 20 minutes on lightly floured surface. Cut each 12-inch square into 16 (3-inch) squares.

2. Preheat air fryer to 360°F.

3. Combine cheese, spinach and pepper in small bowl; mix well.

4. Place about 1 teaspoon cheese mixture in center of each pastry square. Brush edges of squares with water. Bring edges together over filling; twist tightly to seal. Fan out corners of puff pastry.

5. Cook in batches 8 to 10 minutes or until golden brown. Serve warm with sweet and sour sauce, if desired.

*MAKES 32 BUNDLES*

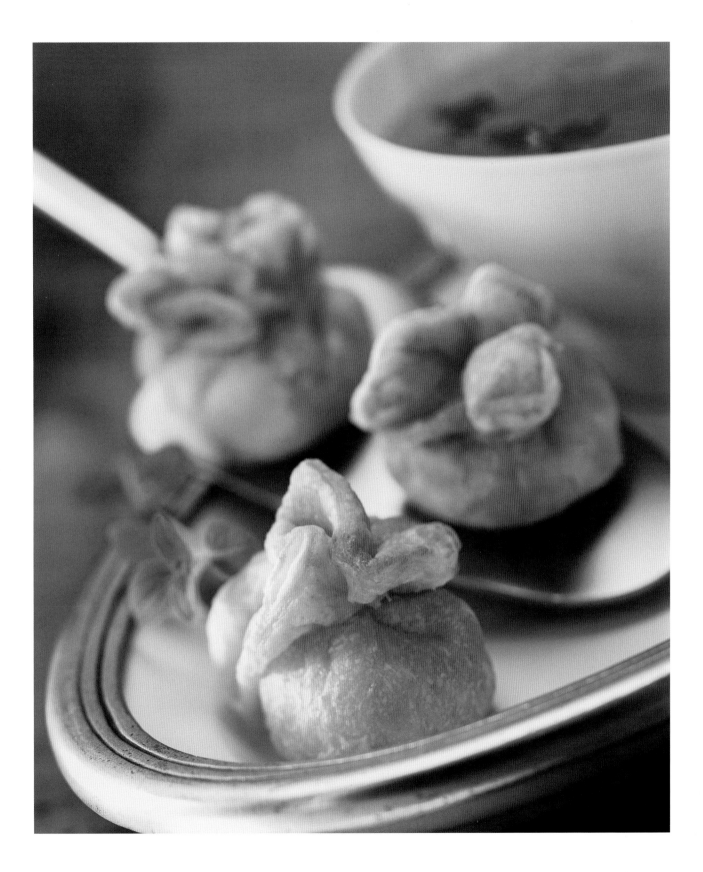

# Avocado Egg Rolls

## DIPPING SAUCE

½ cup cashew nut pieces

½ cup packed fresh cilantro

¼ cup honey

2 green onions, coarsely chopped

2 cloves garlic

1 tablespoon white vinegar

1 teaspoon balsamic vinegar

1 teaspoon ground cumin

½ teaspoon tamarind paste

⅛ teaspoon ground turmeric

¼ cup olive oil

## EGG ROLLS

2 avocados, peeled and pitted

¼ cup chopped drained oil-packed sun-dried tomatoes

2 tablespoons diced red onion

2 tablespoons chopped fresh cilantro

1 tablespoon lime juice

¼ teaspoon salt

10 egg roll wrappers

1 tablespoon vegetable oil

1. For sauce, combine cashews, cilantro, honey, green onions, garlic, white vinegar, balsamic vinegar, cumin, tamarind paste and turmeric in food processor; process until coarsely chopped. With motor running, drizzle in olive oil in thin, steady stream; process until finely chopped and well blended. Refrigerate until ready to use.

2. For egg rolls, place avocados in medium bowl; coarsely mash with potato masher. Stir in sun-dried tomatoes, red onion, chopped cilantro, lime juice and salt until well blended.

3. Working with one at a time, place egg roll wrapper on work surface with one corner facing you. Spread 2 tablespoons filling horizontally across wrapper. Fold short sides over filling and fold up bottom corner over filling. Moisten top edges with water; roll up egg roll, pressing to seal. Refrigerate until ready to cook.

4. Preheat air fryer to 390°F. Brush egg rolls with vegetable oil.

5. Cook in batches 6 to 8 minutes or until golden brown and crispy, turning once. Cut egg rolls in half diagonally; serve with sauce.

*MAKES 8 TO 10 SERVINGS (20 PIECES)*
*AND 1 CUP SAUCE*

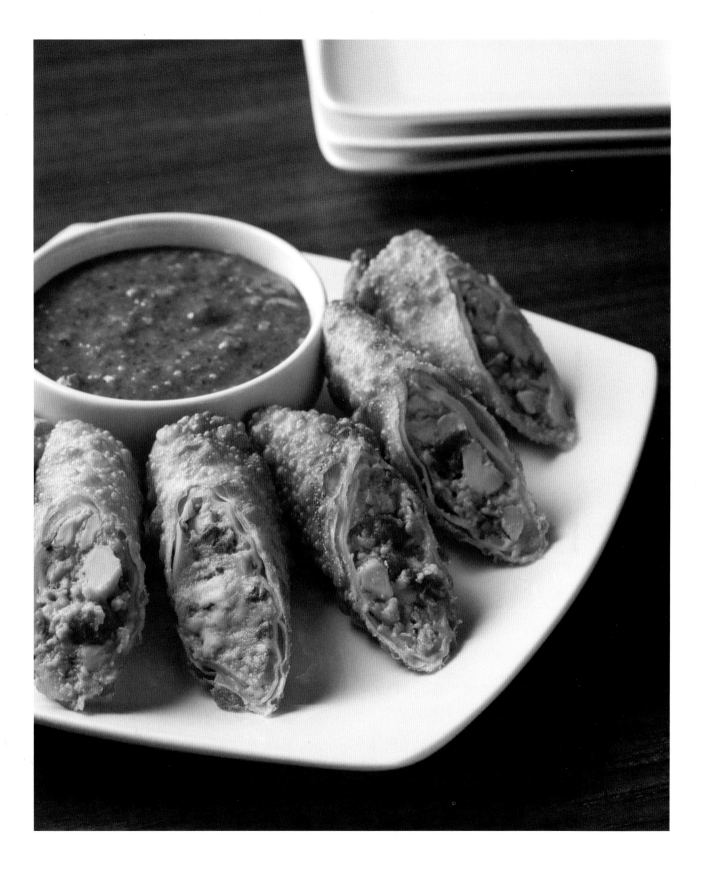

# Cheese & Sausage Bundles

¼ pound bulk hot Italian pork sausage

1 cup (4 ounces) shredded Monterey Jack cheese

1 can (4 ounces) diced mild green chiles, drained

2 tablespoons finely chopped green onion

40 wonton wrappers

Prepared salsa

1. Brown sausage in small skillet over medium-high heat 6 to 8 minutes, stirring to separate meat. Drain off drippings.

2. Combine sausage, cheese, chilies and green onion in medium bowl. Spoon 1 round teaspoon sausage mixture near one corner of wonton wrapper. Brush opposite corner with water. Fold corner over filling; roll into cylinder.

3. Moisten ends of roll with water. Bring ends together to make a "bundle," overlapping ends slightly; firmly press to seal. Repeat with remaining filling and wonton wrappers.

4. Preheat air fryer to 370°F. Cook in batches 3 to 5 minutes or until golden brown. Serve with salsa.

*MAKES 40 APPETIZERS*

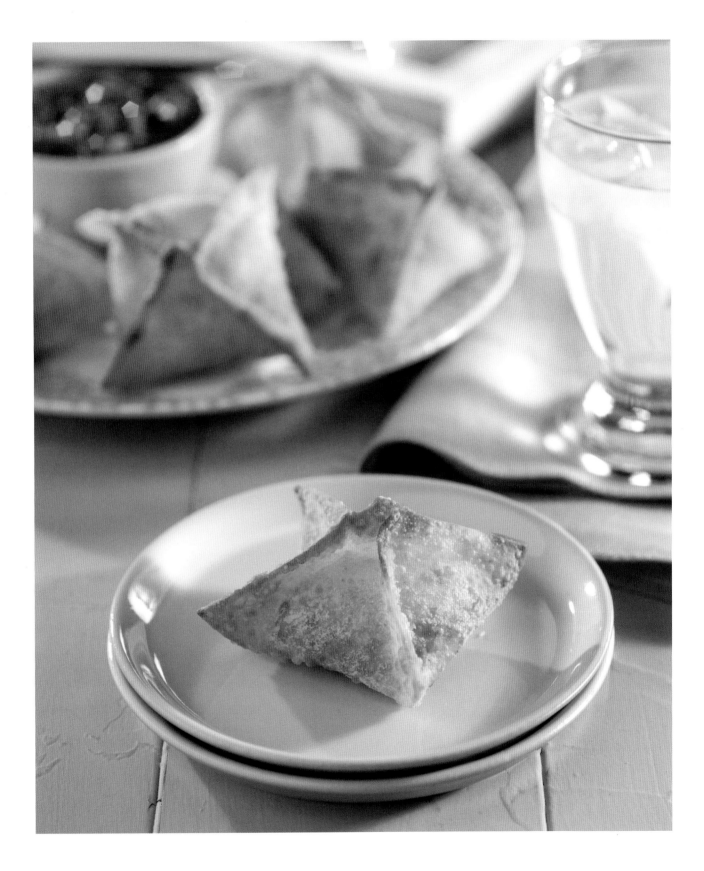

# Coconut Shrimp with Pear Chutney

Pear Chutney
(recipe follows)

½ cup shredded unsweetened
  coconut

¾ teaspoon curry powder

½ teaspoon salt

1 pound large raw shrimp, peeled
  and deveined (with tails on)

3 tablespoons melted unsalted
  butter

1. Prepare Pear Chutney; set aside. Preheat air fryer to 350°F. Spray air fryer basket with nonstick cooking spray.

2. Combine coconut, curry powder and salt in shallow dish. Toss shrimp with melted butter to coat. Dip shrimp in coconut mixture, pressing lightly to adhere.

3. Cook in batches 10 to 12 minutes, turning once halfway through cooking until shrimp are pink and opaque. Serve with Pear Chutney.

*MAKES 4 SERVINGS*

# Pear Chutney

1 tablespoon vegetable oil

1 jalapeño pepper,* seeded and
  minced

1 small shallot, minced

1 teaspoon grated fresh ginger

1 medium unpeeled ripe pear, cored
  and cut into ½-inch pieces

2 teaspoons cider vinegar

1 teaspoon packed brown sugar

⅛ teaspoon salt

1 to 2 tablespoons water

1 tablespoon chopped green onion

*Jalapeño peppers can sting and irritate the skin, so wear rubber gloves when handling peppers and do not touch your eyes.*

1. Heat oil in medium saucepan over low heat. Add jalapeño pepper, shallot and ginger; cook and stir 3 minutes or until shallot is tender.

2. Add pear, vinegar, brown sugar and salt. Stir in 1 tablespoon water. Cover; cook over low heat 15 minutes or until pear is tender, adding additional 1 tablespoon water if mixture becomes dry. Stir in green onion; cook 1 minute. Let cool before serving.

*MAKES 2 CUPS*

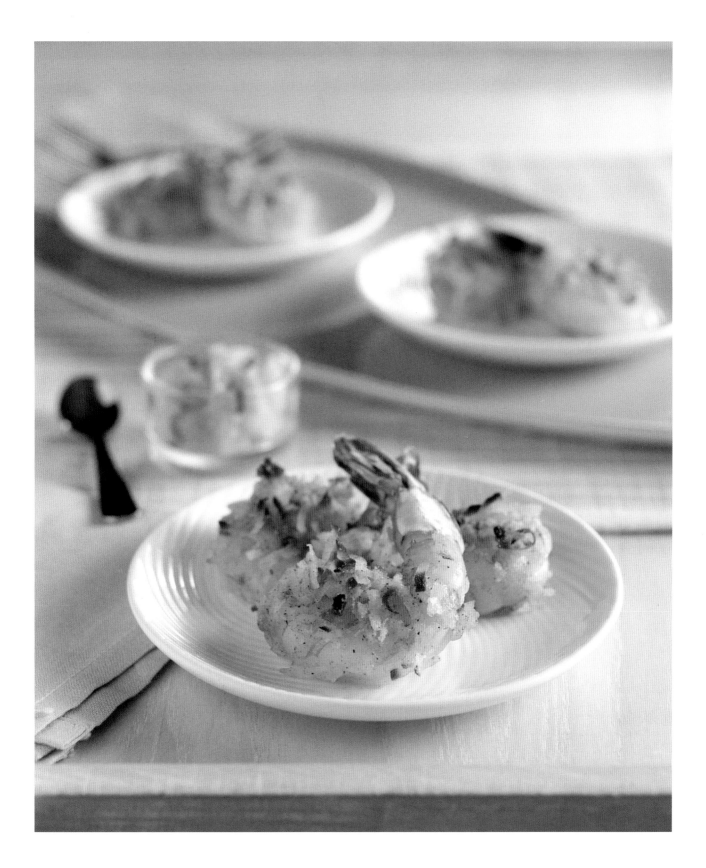

# Brie Bites

1 package (17¼ ounces)
  frozen puff pastry
  (2 sheets)

¼ cup apricot preserves *or* red
  pepper jelly

1 round (8-ounces) Brie, cut
  into 32 cubes

1. Unfold puff pastry; thaw 20 minutes on lightly floured surface.

2. Preheat air fryer to 370°F. Cut each pastry sheet into 16 squares.

3. Spread ½ teaspoon apricot preserves on each square. Place one cube Brie on one side of each square. Fold over opposite edge; use fork to seal edges completely.

4. Cook in batches 8 to 10 minutes or until pastry is golden brown.

*MAKES 32 BITES*

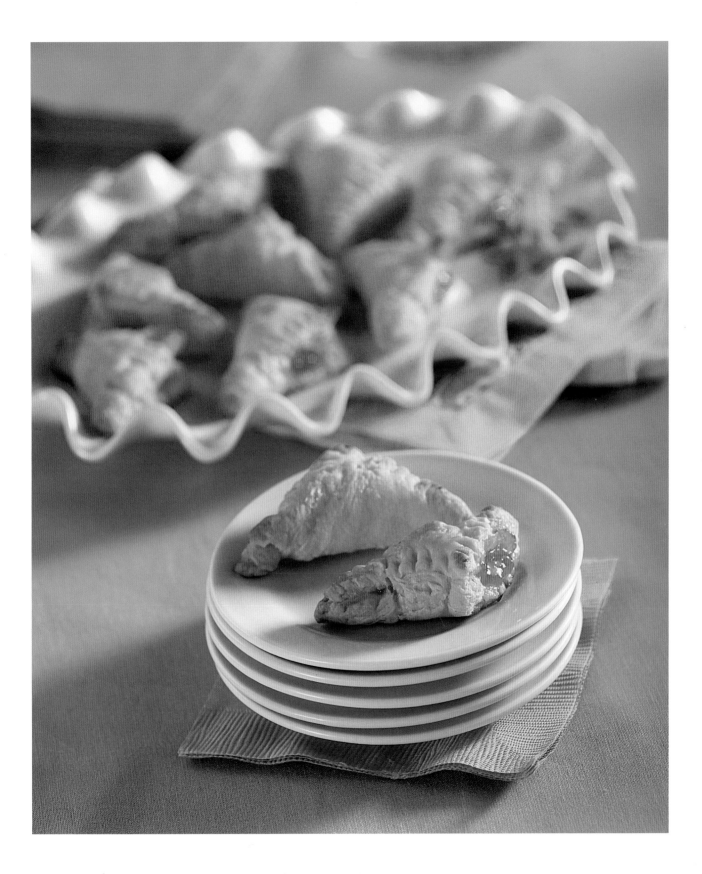

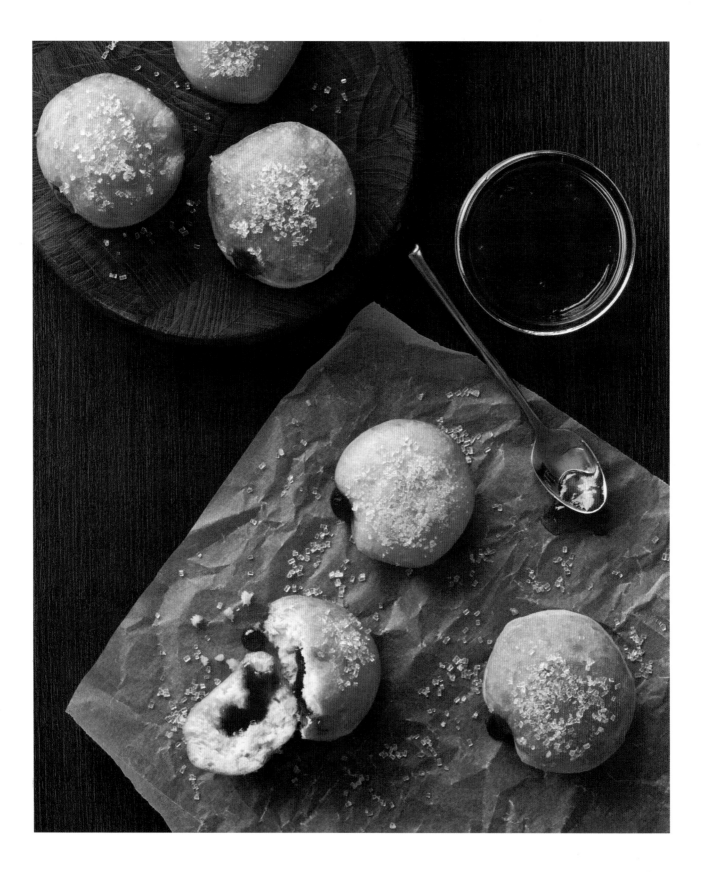

# Breads & Breakfast

# Breakfast Flats

1 package (14 ounces) refrigerated pizza dough

All-purpose flour, for dusting

1½ cups (6 ounces) shredded medium Cheddar cheese

8 slices bacon, cooked crisp and diced

4 eggs, fried

Kosher salt and black pepper (optional)

1. Preheat air fryer to 370°F. Line air fryer basket with parchment paper.

2. Divide pizza dough into four equal portions. Roll out on lightly floured surface into rectangles roughly 8½×4 inches. Top each evenly with cheese and bacon. Cook in batches 5 to 7 minutes or until crust is golden brown and crisp and cheese is melted.

3. Top baked flats with fried egg; season with salt and pepper, if desired. Serve warm.

MAKES 4 SERVINGS

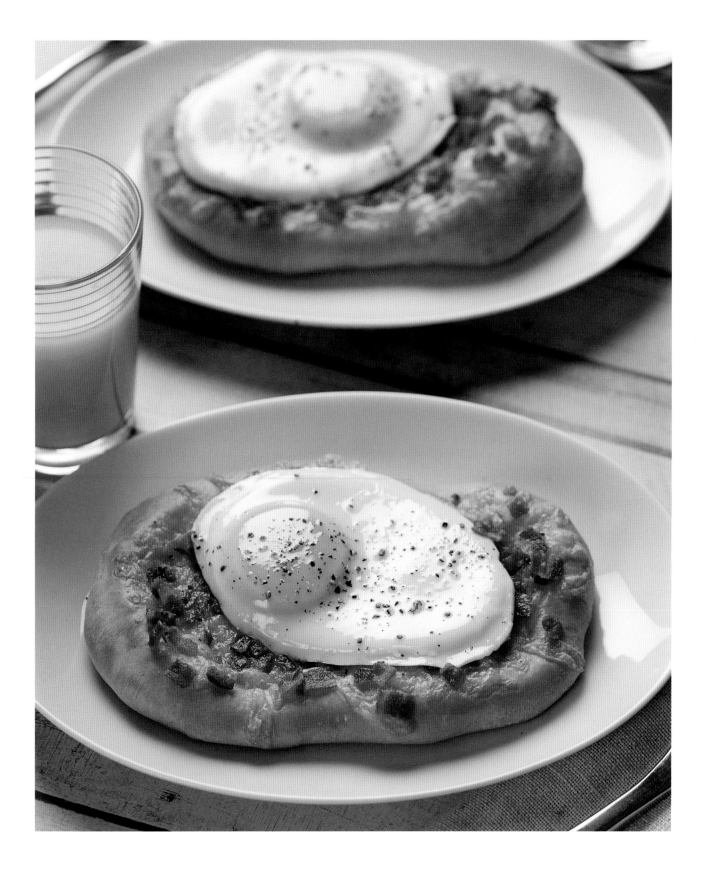

# French Toast Sticks

4 eggs

⅓ cup milk

1 teaspoon ground cinnamon

1 teaspoon vanilla

4 slices thick-cut bread, cut into 3 portions each

1 teaspoon powdered sugar

¼ cup maple syrup

1. Combine eggs, milk, cinnamon and vanilla in large bowl.

2. Dip bread sticks in egg mixture to coat.

3. Preheat air fryer to 370°F. Line air fryer basket with parchment paper; spray with nonstick cooking spray.

4. Cook in batches 8 to 10 minutes or until golden brown. Dust lightly with powdered sugar; serve with syrup.

*MAKES 4 SERVINGS*

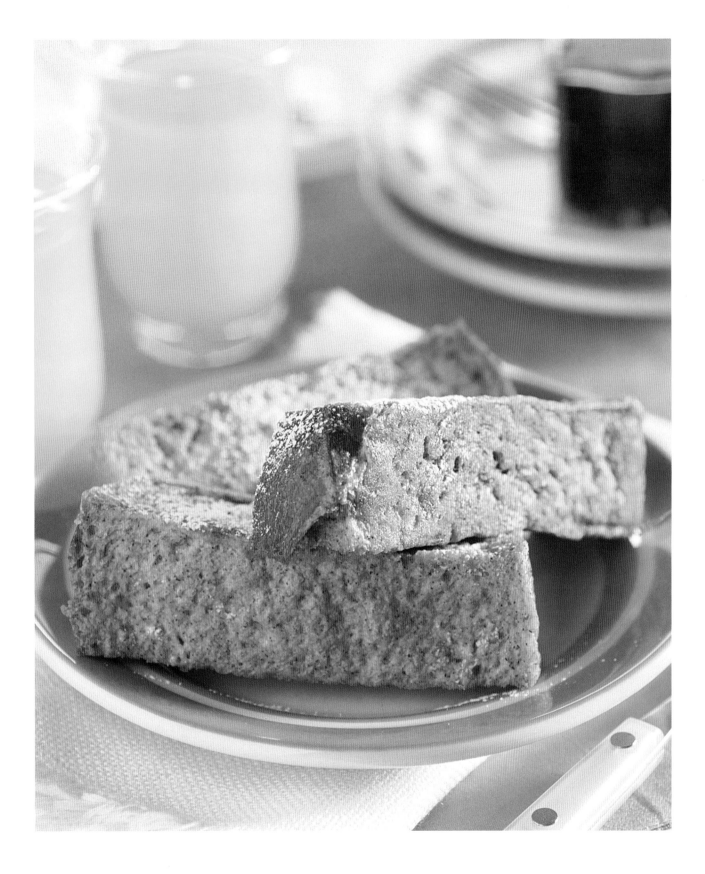

# Lemon Poppy Seed Muffins

2 cups all-purpose flour

1¼ cups granulated sugar

¼ cup poppy seeds

2 tablespoons plus
  2 teaspoons grated
  lemon peel, divided

2 teaspoons baking powder

½ teaspoon baking soda

½ teaspoon ground cardamom

¼ teaspoon salt

2 eggs

½ cup (1 stick) butter, melted

½ cup milk

½ cup plus 2 tablespoons
  lemon juice, divided

1 cup powdered sugar

1. Preheat air fryer to 350°F. Spray silicon muffin cups with nonstick cooking spray.

2. Combine flour, granulated sugar, poppy seeds, 2 tablespoons lemon peel, baking powder, baking soda, cardamom and salt in large bowl. Beat eggs in medium bowl. Add butter, milk and ½ cup lemon juice; mix well. Add egg mixture to flour mixture; stir just until blended. Spoon batter evenly into prepared muffin cups, filling one-half to three-fourths full.

3. Cook in batches 10 to 12 minutes or until toothpick inserted into centers comes out clean. Cool slightly before removing.

4. Meanwhile, prepare glaze. Combine powdered sugar and remaining 2 teaspoons lemon peel in small bowl; stir in enough remaining lemon juice to make pourable glaze. Place muffins on sheet of foil or waxed paper; drizzle with glaze. Serve warm or at room temperature.

*MAKES 18 MUFFINS*

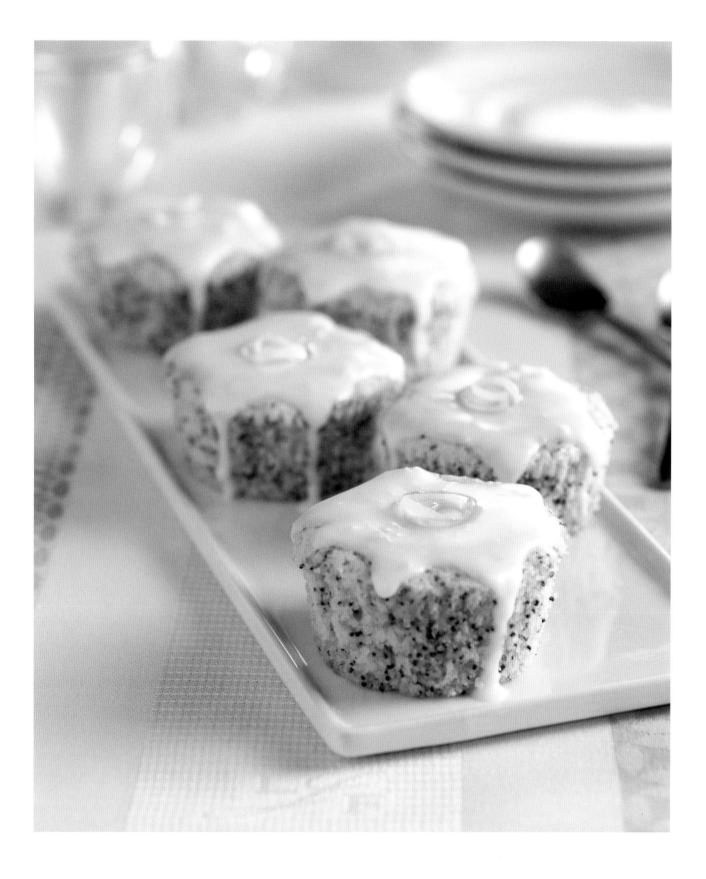

# Quick Jelly-Filled
# Biscuit Doughnut Balls

1 can (about 7 ounces)
   refrigerated biscuit dough
   (10 biscuits)

⅓ cup granulated sugar

1 cup strawberry preserves*

*If preserves are very chunky,
process in food processor 10 seconds
or press through fine-mesh sieve.

1. Preheat air fryer to 370°F.

2. Separate biscuits into 10 portions. Cut each in half; roll dough into balls to create 20 balls.

3. Cook in batches 5 to 6 minutes or until golden brown.

4. Place sugar in large bowl. Coat warm balls in sugar. Let cool. Using a piping bag with medium star tip; fill bag with preserves. Poke hole in side of each doughnut ball with paring knife; fill with preserves. Serve immediately.

*MAKES 20 DOUGHNUT BALLS*

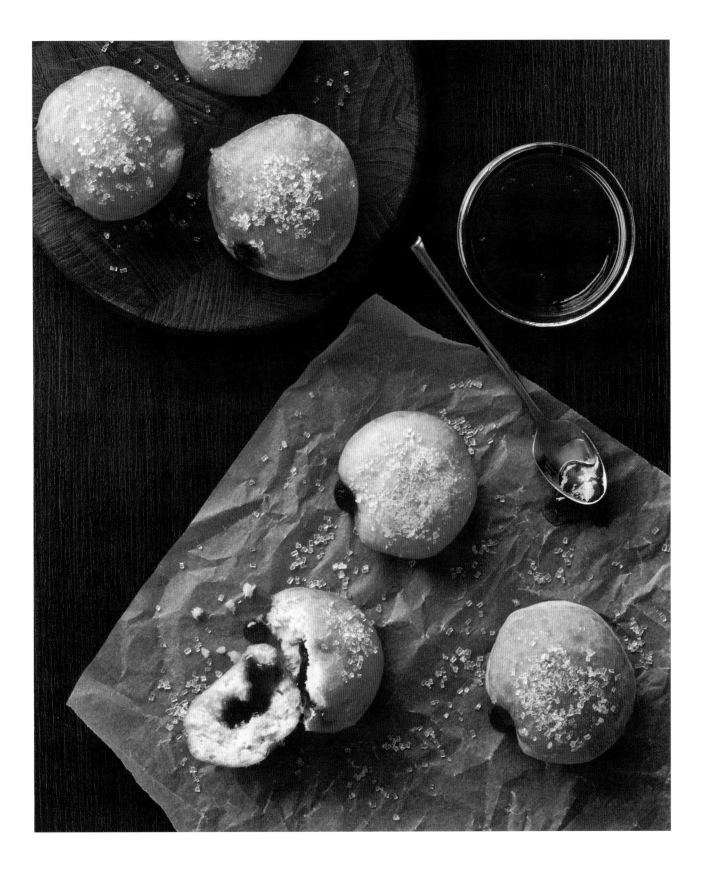

# Breakfast Empanadas

1 package (15 ounces) refrigerated pie crusts (2 crusts)

9 eggs, divided

1 teaspoon water

1 teaspoon salt

Dash black pepper

1 tablespoon butter

½ pound bacon (about 10 slices), crisp-cooked and cut into ¼-inch pieces

2 cups (8 ounces) Mexican-style shredded cheese, divided

4 tablespoons salsa

1. Preheat air fryer to 370°F. Spray air fryer basket with nonstick cooking spray.

2. Place pie crusts on flat surface; cut into halves to make four semicircles.

3. Beat 1 egg and water in small bowl until well blended; set aside. Beat remaining 8 eggs, salt and pepper in medium bowl until well blended. Heat large skillet over medium heat. Add butter; tilt skillet to coat bottom. Sprinkle bacon evenly in skillet. Pour eggs into skillet and cook 2 minutes without stirring. Gently start stirring until eggs form large curds and are still slightly moist. Transfer to plate to cool.

4. Spoon one fourth of cooled scrambled egg mixture onto half of each pie crust. Reserve ¼ cup cheese; sprinkle remaining cheese evenly over eggs. Top with salsa.

5. Brush inside edges of each semicircle with reserved egg-water mixture. Fold dough over top of egg mixture and seal edges with fork. (Flour fork tines to prevent sticking, if necessary.) Brush tops of empanadas with remaining egg-water mixture and sprinkle with reserved ¼ cup cheese.

6. Cook in batches 10 to 12 minutes or until golden.

*MAKES 4 SERVINGS*

Tip: These make a great main dish for dinner, too. Plus, they can be prepared early in the day and reheated in a preheated 350°F oven for 20 to 25 minutes.

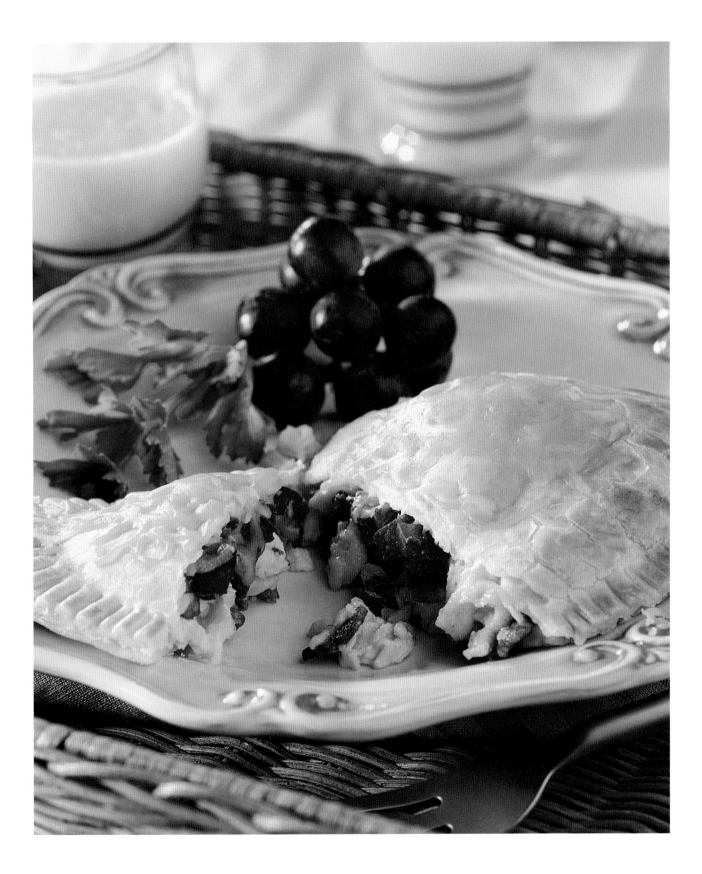

# Bedrock Fruit Boulders

1¼ cups finely chopped apple
(1 small apple)

⅓ cup dried mixed fruit bits

2 tablespoons packed brown
sugar

½ teaspoon ground cinnamon

1 package (about 16 ounces)
refrigerated jumbo
buttermilk biscuits
(8 biscuits)

1 cup sifted powdered sugar

4 to 5 teaspoons orange juice

1. Preheat air fryer to 330°F. Line air fryer basket with parchment paper; spray with nonstick cooking spray.

2. Combine apple, dried fruit, brown sugar and cinnamon in small bowl; mix well.

3. Separate biscuits; cut each biscuit in half horizontally to create 16 rounds. Roll each round into 3½-inch circle. Spoon 1 rounded tablespoon apple mixture into center of each circle. Moisten edges of dough with water. Pull dough up and around filling, completely enclosing filling. Pinch edges to seal. Place seam side down in air fryer basket.

4. Cook in batches 10 to 12 minutes or until golden brown. Cool on wire rack 10 minutes.

5. Combine powdered sugar and 4 teaspoons orange juice in small bowl; whisk until smooth. Add additional orange juice, if necessary, to reach drizzling consistency. Spoon glaze over rolls. Serve warm.

*MAKES 16 SERVINGS*

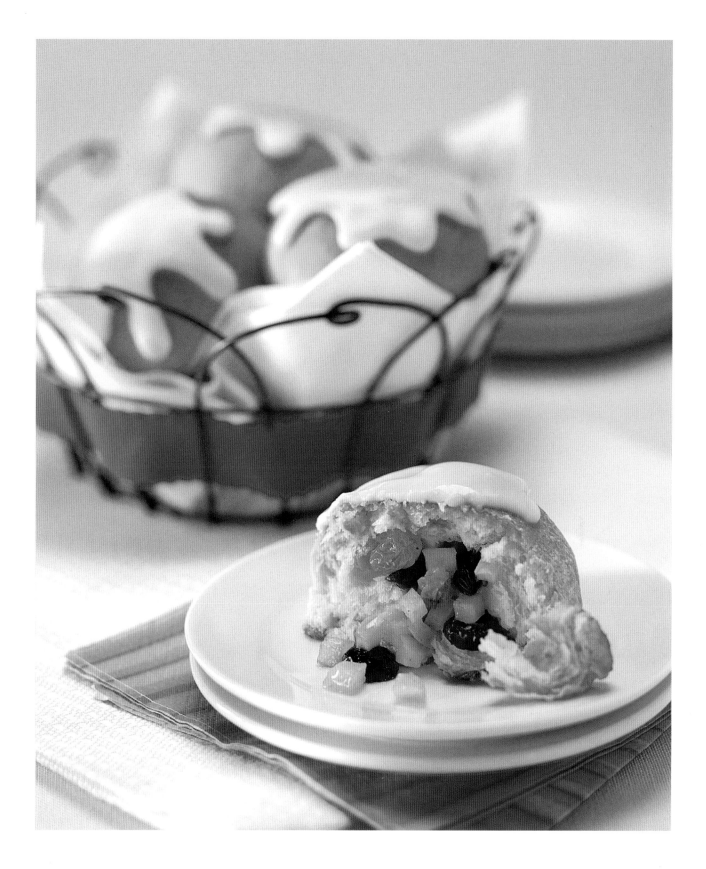

# Crunchy French Toast Sticks

6 slices Italian bread (each 1 inch thick, about 3½ to 4 inches in diameter)

4 cups cornflakes, crushed

3 eggs

⅔ cup milk

1 tablespoon sugar

1 teaspoon ground cinnamon

1 teaspoon vanilla

¼ teaspoon ground nutmeg

1 container (6 ounces) vanilla yogurt

¼ cup maple syrup

Ground cinnamon (optional)

1. Preheat air fryer to 360°F. Remove crusts from bread, if desired. Cut each bread slice into three strips. Place cornflakes on waxed paper.

2. Whisk eggs, milk, sugar, 1 teaspoon cinnamon, vanilla and nutmeg in shallow bowl. Dip bread strips in egg mixture, turning to generously coat all sides. Roll in cornflakes, coating all sides.

3. Cook in batches 18 to 20 minutes or until golden brown, turning sticks after 10 minutes.

4. Meanwhile, combine yogurt and syrup in small bowl. Sprinkle with additional cinnamon, if desired. Serve French toast sticks with yogurt mixture.

*MAKES 6 SERVINGS*

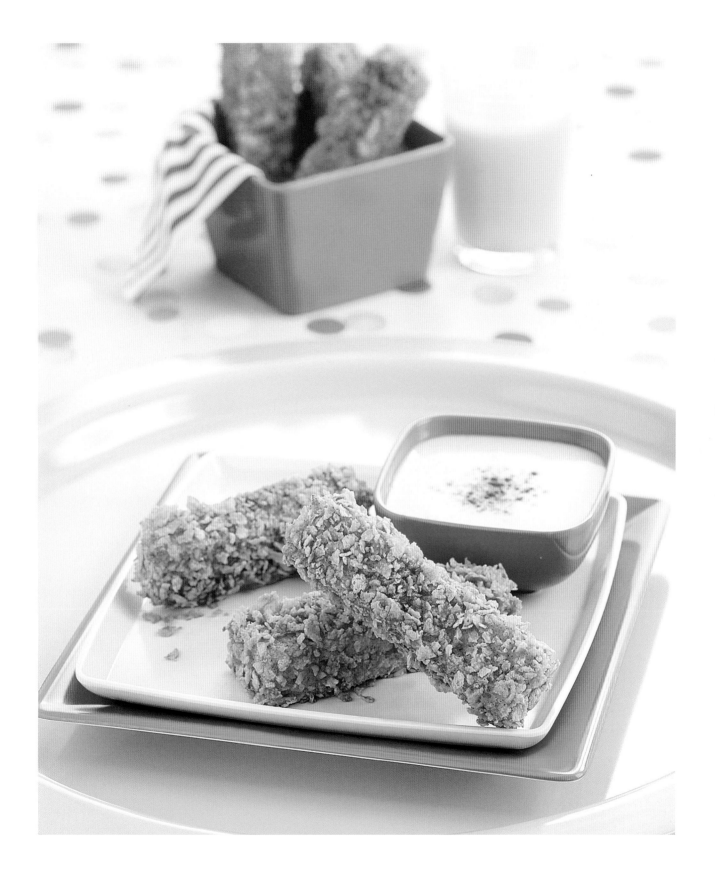

# Biscuit Doughnuts

1 can (about 16 ounces)
   refrigerated jumbo biscuit
   dough (8 biscuits)

¼ cup honey

1 teaspoon chopped
   pistachio nuts

1. Separate dough into 8 portions. Using hands, create a hole in the middle to create doughnut shape.

2. Preheat air fryer to 370°F.

3. Cook in batches 7 to 8 minutes or until golden brown.

4. Drizzle warm doughnuts with honey. Sprinkle with pistachios.

*MAKES 8 DOUGHNUTS*

**Variation:** For cinnamon-sugar coating, combine ¼ cup sugar and 1 teaspoon ground cinnamon in small bowl. Dip warm doughnuts in cinnamon-sugar topping while warm.

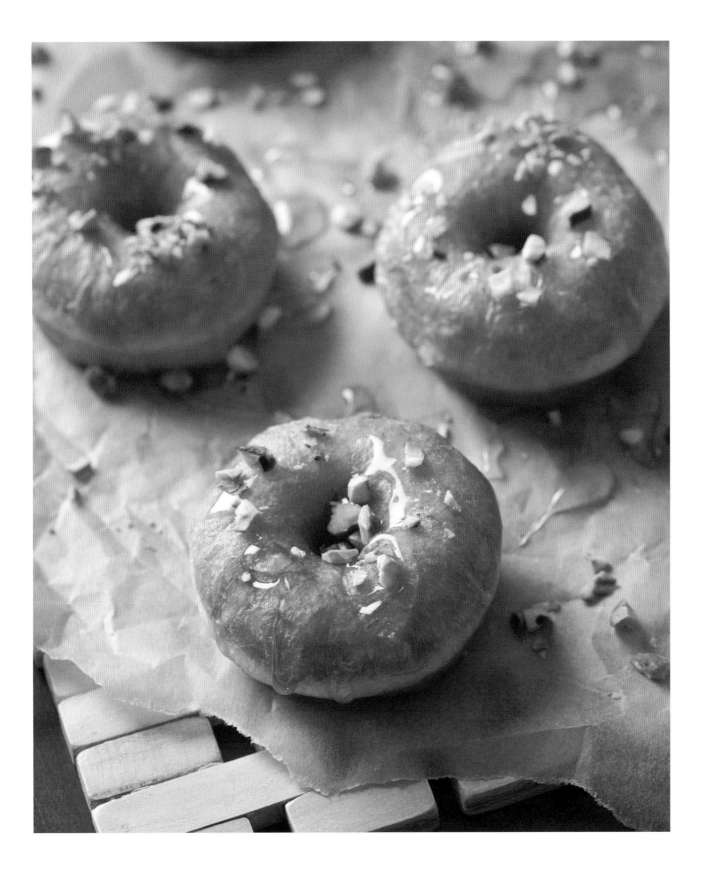

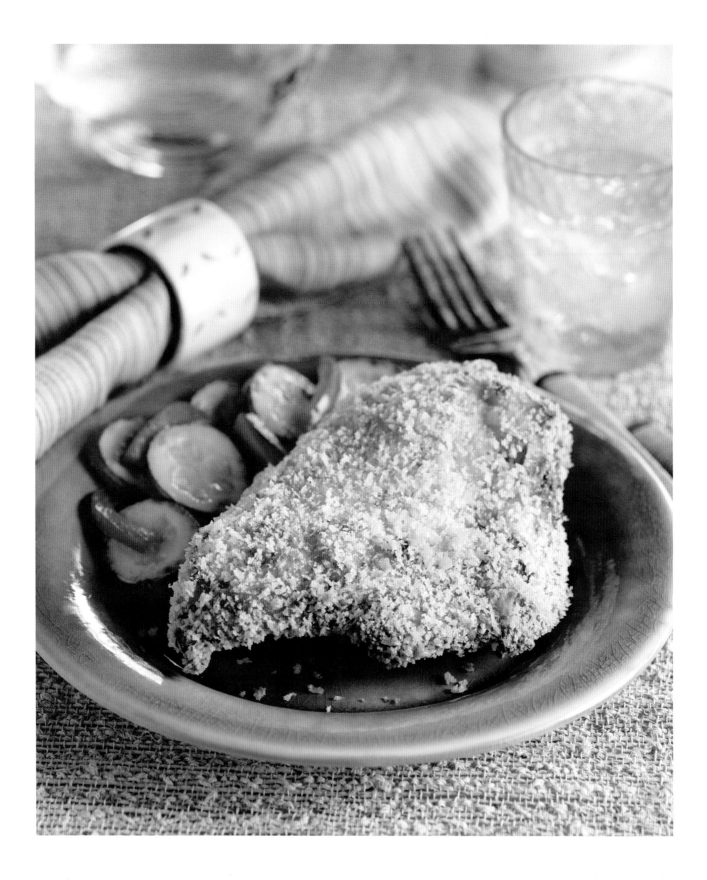

# Easy Dinners

# Breaded Veal Scallopini with Mushrooms

½ pound veal cutlets

½ teaspoon salt, divided

¼ teaspoon black pepper, divided

1 egg

1 tablespoon milk or water

½ cup plain dry bread crumbs

3 tablespoons unsalted butter

2 large shallots, chopped (about ¼ cup)

8 ounces exotic mushrooms, such as cremini, oyster, baby bella and shiitake*

½ teaspoon herbes de Provence**

½ cup reduced-sodium chicken broth

2 lemon wedges (optional)

*Exotic mushrooms make this dish special. However, you can substitute white button mushrooms, if you prefer.

**Herbes de Provence is a mixture of basil, fennel, lavender, marjoram, rosemary, sage, savory and thyme used to season meat, poultry and vegetables.

1. Season cutlets with ¼ teaspoon salt and ⅛ teaspoon pepper. Lightly beat egg with milk in shallow dish. Place bread crumbs in separate shallow dish.

2. Dip cutlet into egg, letting excess drip off. Dip in crumbs, turning to coat. Repeat with remaining cutlets.

3. Preheat air fryer to 370°F. Spray air fryer basket with nonstick cooking spray. Cook cutlets 12 to 15 minutes, turning halfway, until golden brown and cooked through. Transfer to plate.

4. Heat butter in large medium skillet over medium-high heat. Add shallots; cook and stir 1 to 2 minutes or until translucent. Add mushrooms, remaining ¼ teaspoon salt, ⅛ teaspoon pepper and herbes de Provence; cook and stir 3 to 4 minutes or until most of liquid is evaporated. Stir in broth; cook 2 to 3 minutes or until slightly thickened.

5. Pour mushroom mixture over cutlets. Garnish with lemon wedges.

MAKES 2 SERVINGS

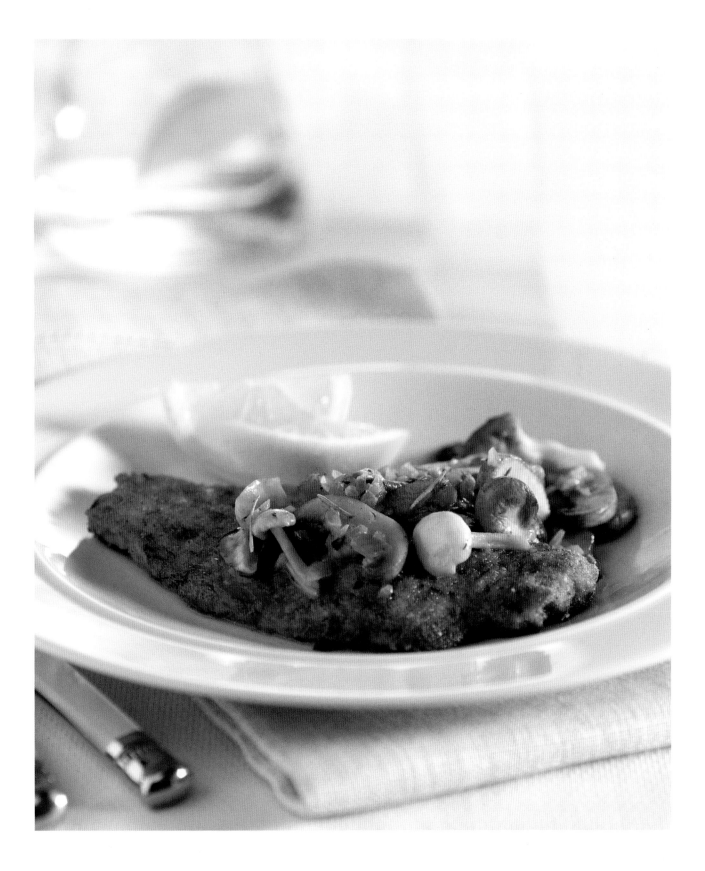

# Salmon-Potato Cakes
# with Mustard Tartar Sauce

3 small unpeeled red potatoes (8 ounces), halved

1 cup water

1 cup flaked cooked salmon

2 green onions, chopped

1 egg white

2 tablespoons chopped fresh parsley, divided

½ teaspoon Cajun or Creole seasoning mix

1 tablespoon mayonnaise

1 tablespoon plain yogurt or sour cream

2 teaspoons coarse-grain mustard

1 tablespoon chopped dill pickle

1 teaspoon lemon juice

1. Place potatoes and water in medium saucepan. Bring to a boil. Reduce heat and simmer about 15 minutes or until potatoes are tender. Drain. Mash potatoes with fork, leaving chunky texture.

2. Combine mashed potatoes, salmon, green onions, egg white, 1 tablespoon parsley and seasoning mix in medium bowl.

3. Preheat air fryer to 370°F. Gently shape salmon mixture into 2 patties; flatten slightly. Cook 5 to 6 minutes or until browned and heated through, turning halfway through cooking time.

4. Meanwhile, combine mayonnaise, yogurt, mustard, remaining 1 tablespoon parsley, pickle and lemon juice in small bowl. Serve sauce with cakes.

*MAKES 2 SERVINGS*

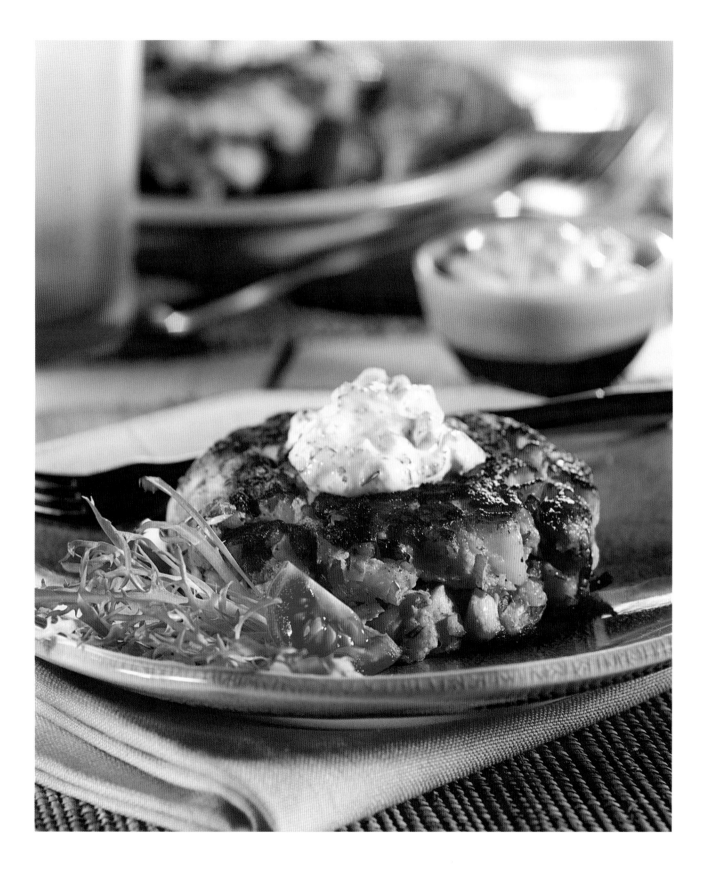

# Beef and Beer Sliders

6 tablespoons ketchup

2 tablespoons mayonnaise

2 teaspoons Dijon mustard

1½ pounds ground beef

½ cup beer

1 teaspoon salt

½ teaspoon garlic powder

½ teaspoon onion powder

½ teaspoon ground cumin

½ teaspoon dried oregano

¼ teaspoon black pepper

3 slices sharp Cheddar cheese, cut into 4 pieces

12 slider buns or potato dinner rolls

12 baby lettuce leaves

12 plum tomato slices

1. Combine ketchup, mayonnaise and mustard in small bowl; reserve.

2. Combine beef, beer, salt, garlic powder, onion powder, cumin, oregano and pepper in medium bowl. Shape mixture into 12 (¼-inch-thick) patties.

3. Preheat air fryer to 370°F. Spray air fryer basket with nonstick cooking spray. Cook patties in batches 6 to 8 minutes; flip over. Top each with 1 piece cheese. Cook in batches 2 to 4 minutes or until cheese is melted and patties are cooked through. Remove to large plate; keep warm.

4. Serve sliders on rolls with ketchup mixture, lettuce and tomato.

*MAKES 12 SLIDERS*

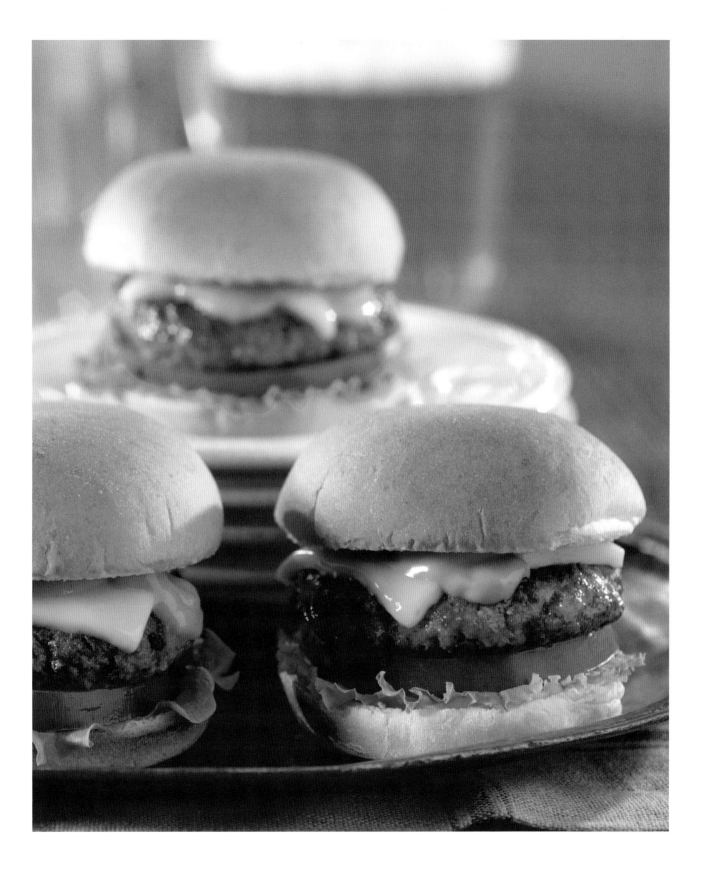

# Teriyaki Salmon

¼ cup sesame oil

Juice of 1 lemon

¼ cup soy sauce

2 tablespoons packed
  brown sugar

1 clove garlic, minced

2 salmon fillets (about
  4 ounces each)

Hot cooked rice

Toasted sesame seeds and
  green onions (optional)

1. Whisk oil, lemon juice, soy sauce, brown sugar and garlic in medium bowl. Place salmon in large resealable food storage bag; add marinade. Refrigerate at least 2 hours.

2. Preheat air fryer to 330°F. Spray air fryer basket with nonstick cooking spray.

3. Cook 8 to 10 minutes until salmon is crispy and easily flakes with a fork. Serve with rice and garnish as desired.

*MAKES 2 SERVINGS*

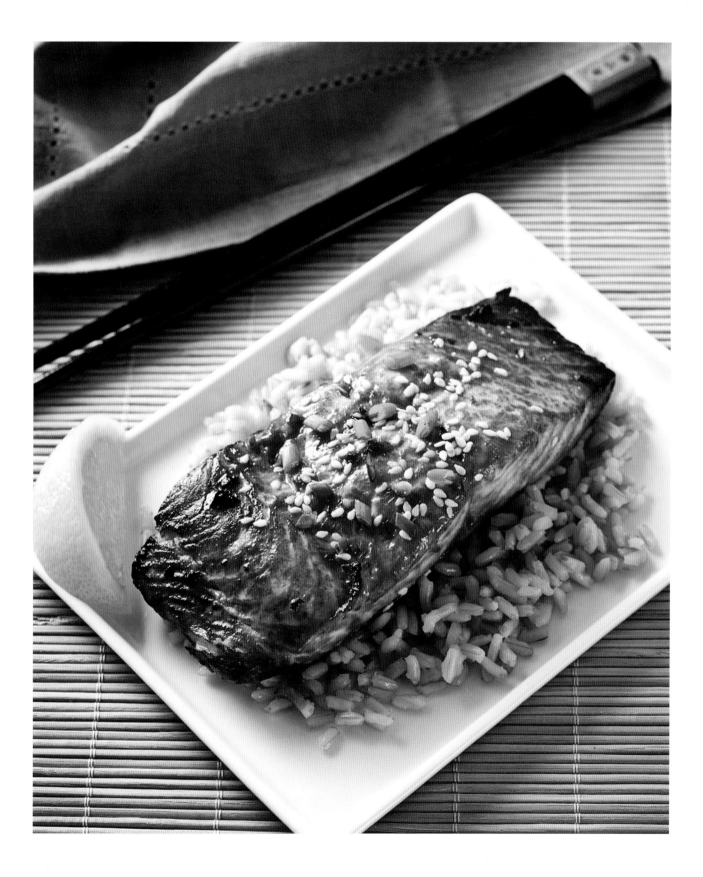

# Baked Pork Buns

1 tablespoon oil

2 cups coarsely chopped
   bok choy

1 small onion or large shallot,
   thinly sliced

1 container (18 ounces)
   refrigerated shredded
   barbecue pork

   All-purpose flour

2 packages (10 ounces
   each) refrigerated jumbo
   buttermilk biscuits
   (5 biscuits per package)

1. Preheat air fryer to 330°F. Line air fryer basket with parchment paper; spray with nonstick cooking spray.

2. Heat oil in large skillet over medium-high heat. Add bok choy and onion; cook and stir 8 to 10 minutes or until vegetables are tender. Remove from heat; stir in barbecue pork.

3. Lightly flour work surface. Separate biscuits; split each biscuit in half to create two thin biscuits. Roll each biscuit half into 5-inch circle.

4. Spoon heaping tablespoon of pork mixture onto one side of each circle. Fold dough over filling to form half circle; press edges to seal.

5. Cook in batches 8 to 10 minutes or until golden brown.

*MAKES 10 BUNS*

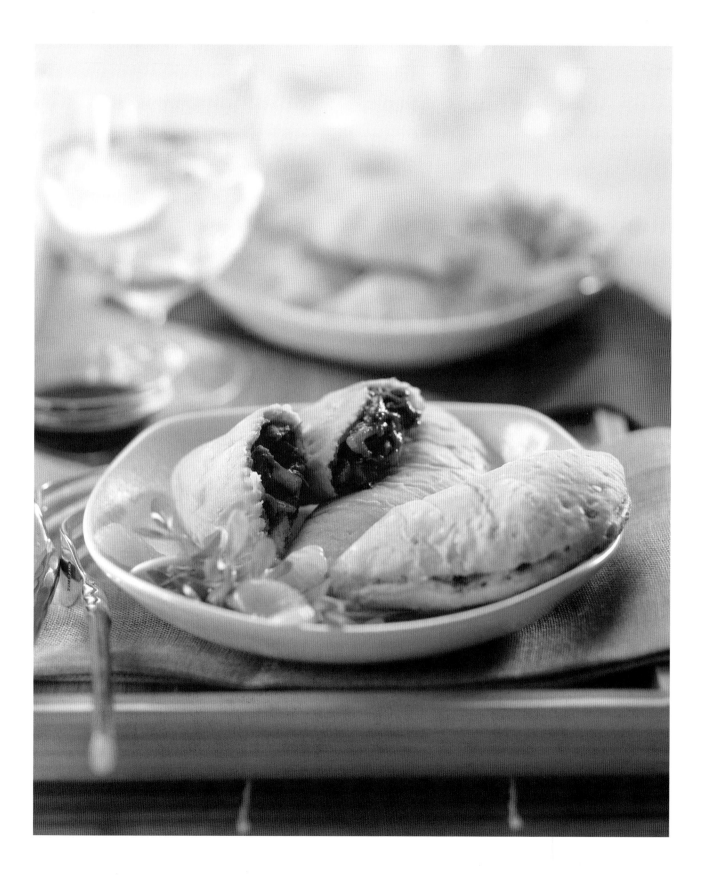

# Blackened Catfish with Easy Tartar Sauce and Rice

Easy Tartar Sauce
(recipe follows)

4  catfish fillets (4 ounces
   each)

2  teaspoons lemon juice

2  teaspoons blackened or
   Cajun seasoning blend

1  cup hot cooked rice
   (optional)

1. Prepare Easy Tartar Sauce.

2. Rinse catfish and pat dry with paper towel. Sprinkle with lemon juice; coat with nonstick cooking spray. Sprinkle with seasoning blend; coat again with cooking spray.

3. Preheat air fryer to 390°F. Cook in batches 8 to 10 minutes, turning halfway through cooking, until fish begins to flake when tested with a fork. Serve with Easy Tartar Sauce and rice.

*MAKES 4 SERVINGS*

# Easy Tartar Sauce

¼  cup mayonnaise

2  tablespoons sweet pickle
   relish

1  teaspoon lemon juice

Combine mayonnaise, relish and lemon juice in small bowl; mix well. Cover and refrigerate until ready to serve.

*MAKES ABOUT ¼ CUP*

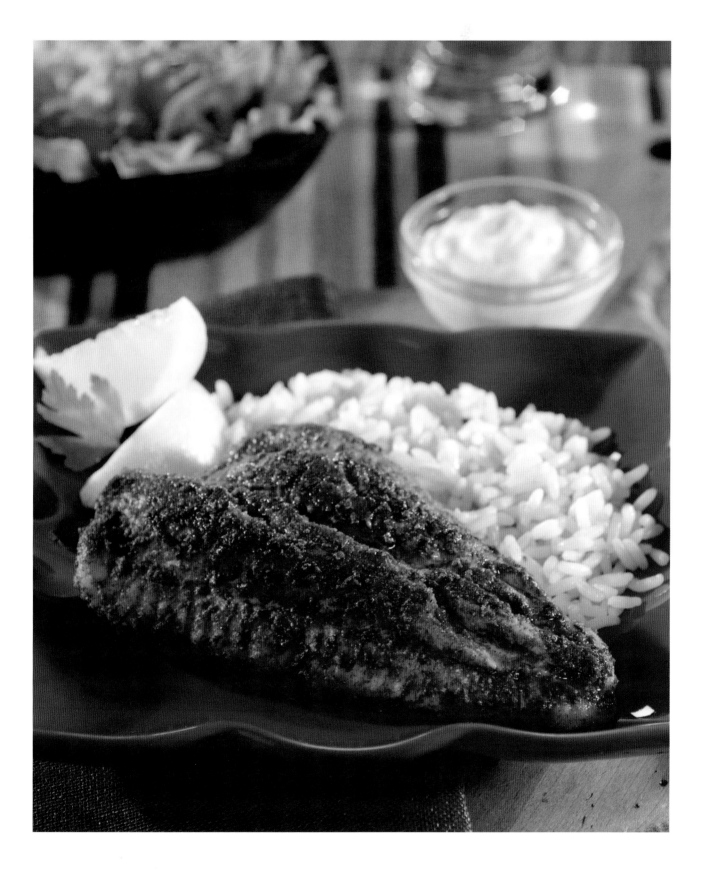

# Blue Cheese Stuffed Chicken Breasts

½ cup crumbled blue cheese

2 tablespoons butter, softened, divided

¾ teaspoon dried thyme

Salt and black pepper

4 bone-in skin-on chicken breasts

1 tablespoon lemon juice

1. Preheat air fryer to 370°F. Combine cheese, 1 tablespoon butter and thyme in small bowl; mix well. Season with salt and pepper.

2. Loosen chicken skin by pushing fingers between skin and meat, taking care not to tear skin. Spread cheese mixture under skin; massage skin to spread mixture evenly over chicken breast.

3. Melt remaining 1 tablespoon butter in small bowl; stir in lemon juice until blended. Brush mixture over chicken. Sprinkle with salt and pepper.

4. Cook 22 to 24 minutes or until chicken is cooked through.

*MAKES 4 SERVINGS*

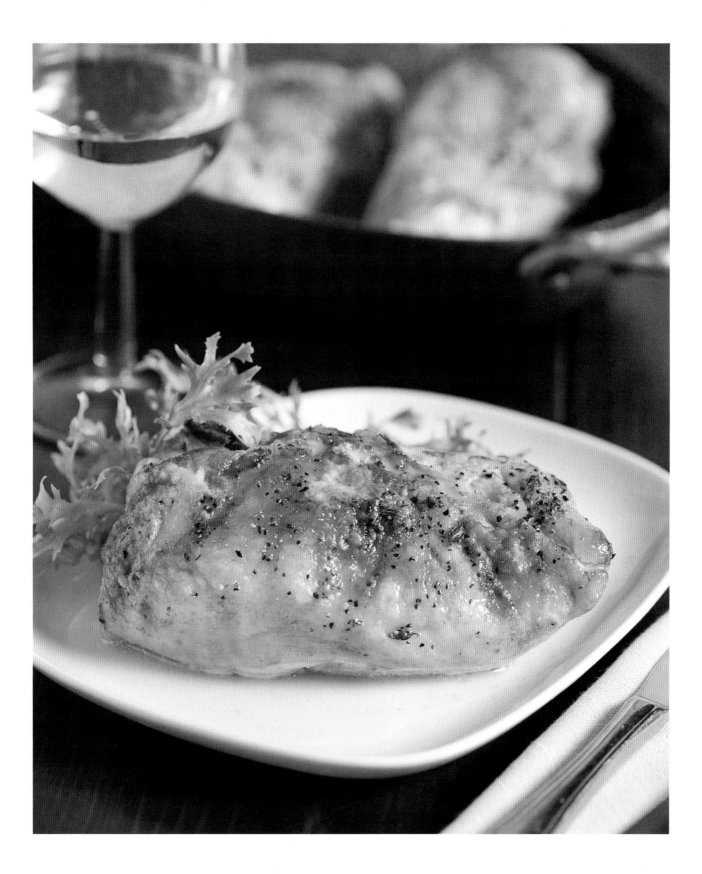

# Vegetable and Hummus Muffaletta

- 1 small eggplant, cut lengthwise into ⅛-inch slices
- 1 yellow squash, cut lengthwise into ⅛-inch slices
- 1 zucchini, cut on the diagonal into ⅛-inch slices
- 1 tablespoon extra virgin olive oil
- ½ teaspoon salt
- ¼ teaspoon black pepper
- 1 (8-inch) boule or round bread, cut in half horizontally
- 1 container (8 ounces) hummus, any flavor
- 1 jar (12 ounces) roasted red bell peppers, drained
- 1 jar (6 ounces) marinated artichoke hearts, drained and chopped
- 1 small tomato, thinly sliced

1. Preheat air fryer to 390°F. Combine eggplant, yellow squash, zucchini, oil, salt and black pepper in large bowl; toss to coat. Cook in batches 4 to 6 minutes per side or until tender and golden. Cool to room temperature.

2. Scoop out bread from both halves of boule, leaving about 1 inch of bread on edges and about 1½ inches on bottom. (Reserve bread for bread crumbs or croutons.) Spread hummus evenly on inside bottom of bread. Layer grilled vegetables, roasted peppers, artichokes and tomato over hummus; cover with top half of bread. Wrap stuffed loaf tightly in plastic wrap. Refrigerate at least 1 hour before cutting into wedges.

*MAKES 6 SERVINGS*

Substitution: You can also roast red bell peppers in the air fryer. Cook 390°F. 15 minutes, turning once or twice. Let sit in air fryer 10 minutes longer to loosen skin. Carefully remove skin with paring knife.

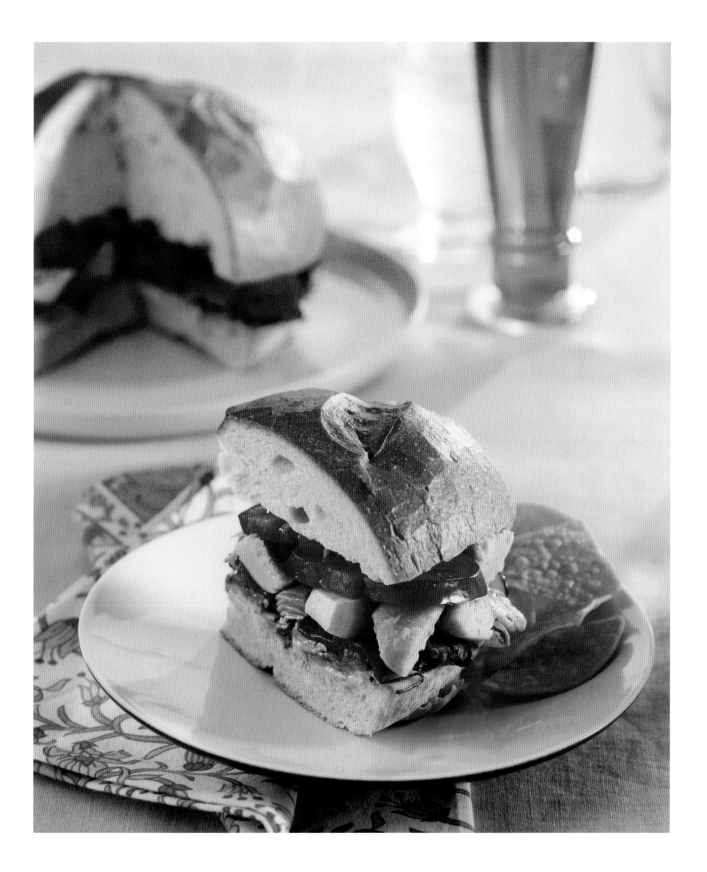

# Buttermilk Air-Fried Chicken

1 cut-up whole chicken
   (2½ to 3 pounds)

1 cup buttermilk

¾ cup all-purpose flour

½ teaspoon salt

½ teaspoon ground red
   pepper

¼ teaspoon garlic powder

2 cups plain dry bread
   crumbs

1. Place chicken pieces in large resealable food storage bag. Pour buttermilk over chicken. Close and refrigerate; let marinate at least 2 hours.

2. Preheat air fryer to 390°F. Spray air fryer basket with nonstick cooking spray.

3. Combine flour, salt, ground red pepper and garlic powder in large shallow bowl. Place bread crumbs in another shallow bowl.

4. Remove chicken pieces from buttermilk; coat with flour mixture then coat in bread crumbs. Spray chicken with cooking spray. Cook 20 to 25 minutes or until brown and crisp on all sides and cooked through (165°F). Serve warm.

*MAKES 4 SERVINGS*

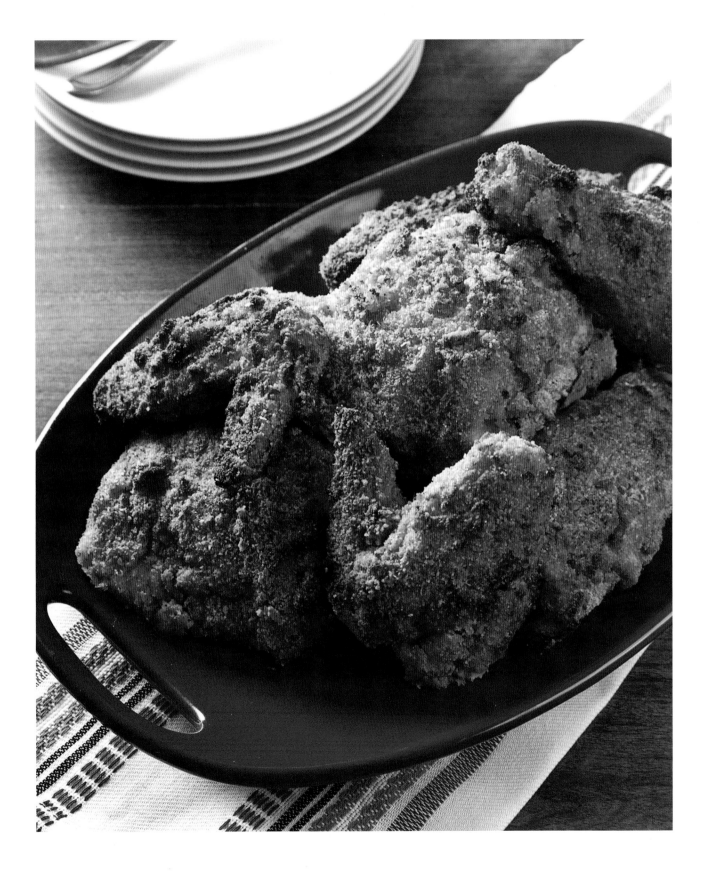

# Coconut Shrimp

## DIPPING SAUCE

½ cup orange marmalade

⅓ cup Thai chili sauce

1 teaspoon prepared
   horseradish

½ teaspoon salt

## SHRIMP

1 cup flat beer

1 cup all-purpose flour

2 cups sweetened flaked
   coconut, divided

2 tablespoons sugar

16 to 20 large raw shrimp,
   peeled and deveined
   (with tails on), patted dry

1. For dipping sauce, combine marmalade, chili sauce, horseradish and salt in small bowl; mix well. Cover and refrigerate until ready to serve.

2. For shrimp, whisk beer, flour, ½ cup coconut and sugar in large bowl until well blended. Place remaining 1½ cups coconut in medium bowl.

3. Preheat air fryer to 390°F. Dip shrimp in beer batter, then in coconut, turning to coat completely. Cook in batches 5 to 7 minutes or until golden brown, turning halfway through cooking. Serve with dipping sauce.

*MAKES 4 SERVINGS*

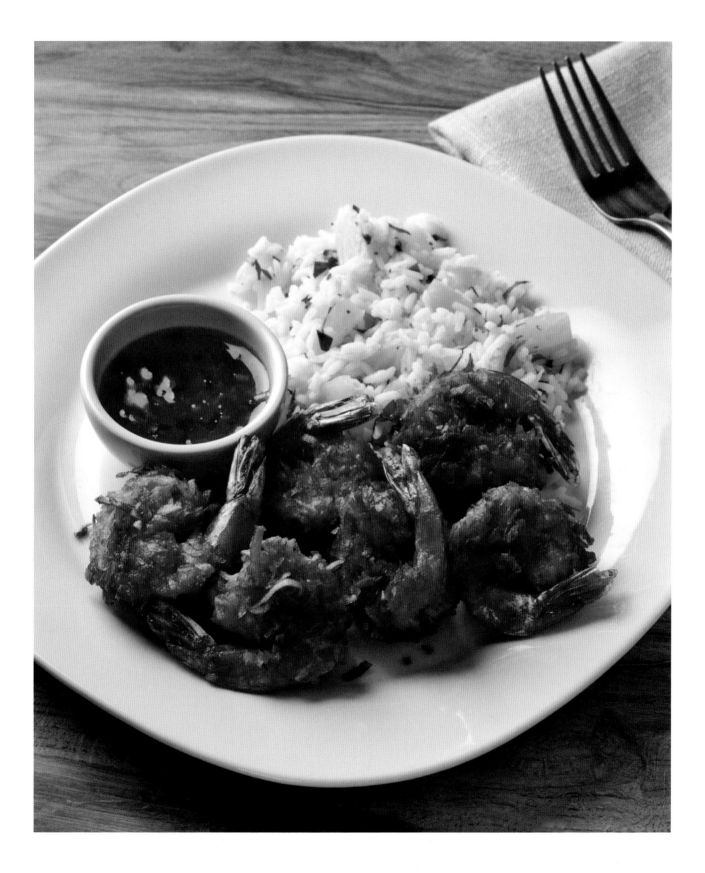

# Beer Air-Fried Chicken

1⅓ cups light-colored beer, such as pale ale

2 tablespoons buttermilk

1¼ cups panko bread crumbs*

½ cup grated Parmesan cheese

4 chicken breast cutlets (about 1¼ pounds)

½ teaspoon salt

¼ teaspoon black pepper

*Panko bread crumbs are used in Japanese cooking to provide a crisp exterior to foods. They are coarser than ordinary bread crumbs. Panko can be found in Asian markets or in the Asian aisle of supermarkets.*

1. Preheat air fryer to 370°F. Line air fryer basket with foil; spray with nonstick cooking spray.

2. Combine beer and buttermilk in shallow bowl. Combine panko and cheese in another shallow bowl.

3. Sprinkle chicken with salt and pepper. Dip in beer mixture; roll in panko mixture to coat.

4. Cook 18 to 20 minutes or until chicken is no longer pink in center.

*MAKES 4 SERVINGS*

**Tip:** To make a substitution for buttermilk, place 1 teaspoon lemon juice or distilled white vinegar in a measuring cup and add enough milk to measure ⅓ cup. Stir and let the mixture stand at room temperature for 5 minutes. Discard leftover mixture.

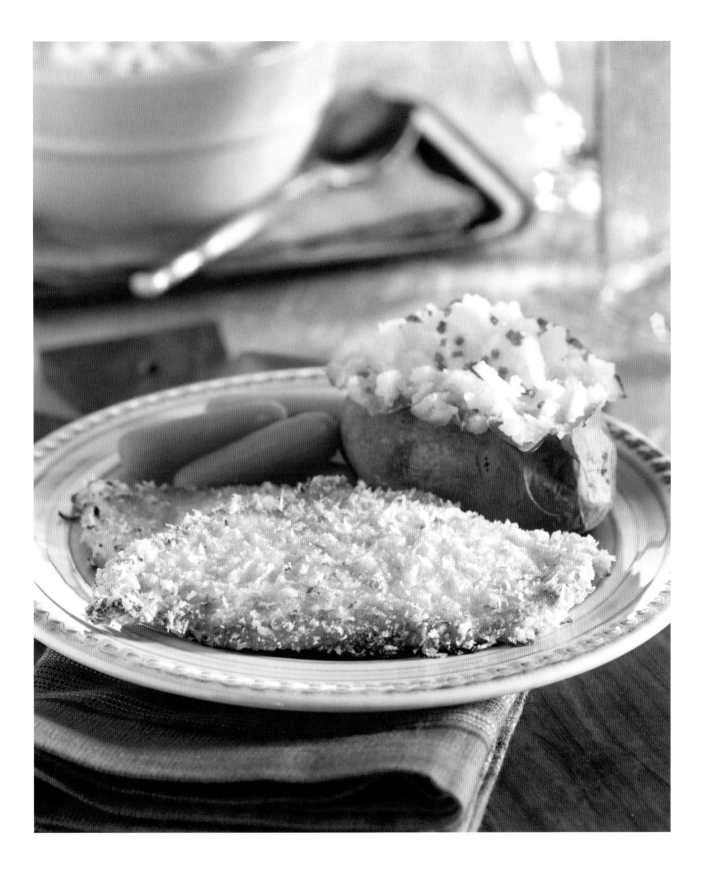

# Chicken Salad with Creamy Tarragon Dressing

Creamy Tarragon Dressing (recipe follows)

1 pound chicken tenders

1 teaspoon Cajun or Creole seasoning*

1 package (10 ounces) mixed salad greens

2 unpeeled apples, cored and thinly sliced

1 cup packed alfalfa sprouts

2 tablespoons raisins

*Adjust your seasoning if your prefer more or less of a spicier taste.*

1. Prepare Creamy Tarragon Dressing. Preheat air fryer to 370°F.

2. Season chicken with Cajun seasoning. Spray chicken with nonstick cooking spray. Cook in batches 10 to 12 minutes or until no longer pink in center.

3. Divide salad greens among four large plates. Arrange chicken, apples and sprouts on top of greens. Sprinkle with raisins. Serve with dressing.

*MAKES 4 SERVINGS*

# Creamy Tarragon Dressing

½ cup plain yogurt

¼ cup sour cream

¼ cup frozen apple juice concentrate

1 tablespoon spicy brown mustard

1 tablespoon minced fresh tarragon leaves

Combine all ingredients in small bowl.

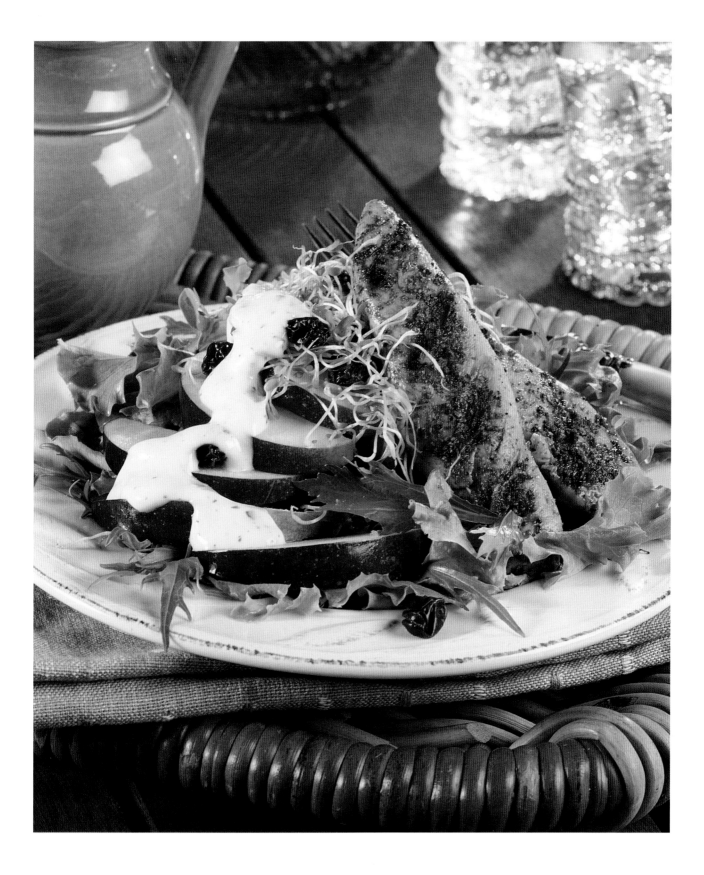

# Buffalo Chicken Wraps

2 boneless skinless chicken breasts (about 4 ounces each)

¼ cup buffalo wing sauce, divided

1 cup broccoli slaw

1½ teaspoons light blue cheese salad dressing

2 (8-inch) whole wheat tortillas, warmed

1. Place chicken in large resealable food storage bag. Add 2 tablespoons buffalo sauce; seal bag. Marinate in refrigerator 15 minutes.

2. Meanwhile, preheat air fryer to 390°F. Cook 8 to 10 minutes per side or until no longer pink. When cool enough to handle, slice chicken; combine with remaining 2 tablespoons buffalo sauce in medium bowl.

3. Combine broccoli slaw and blue cheese dressing in medium bowl; mix well.

4. Arrange chicken and broccoli slaw evenly down center of each tortilla. Roll up to secure filling. To serve, cut in half diagonally.

*MAKES 2 SERVINGS*

Tip: If you don't like the spicy flavor of buffalo wing sauce, substitute your favorite barbecue sauce.

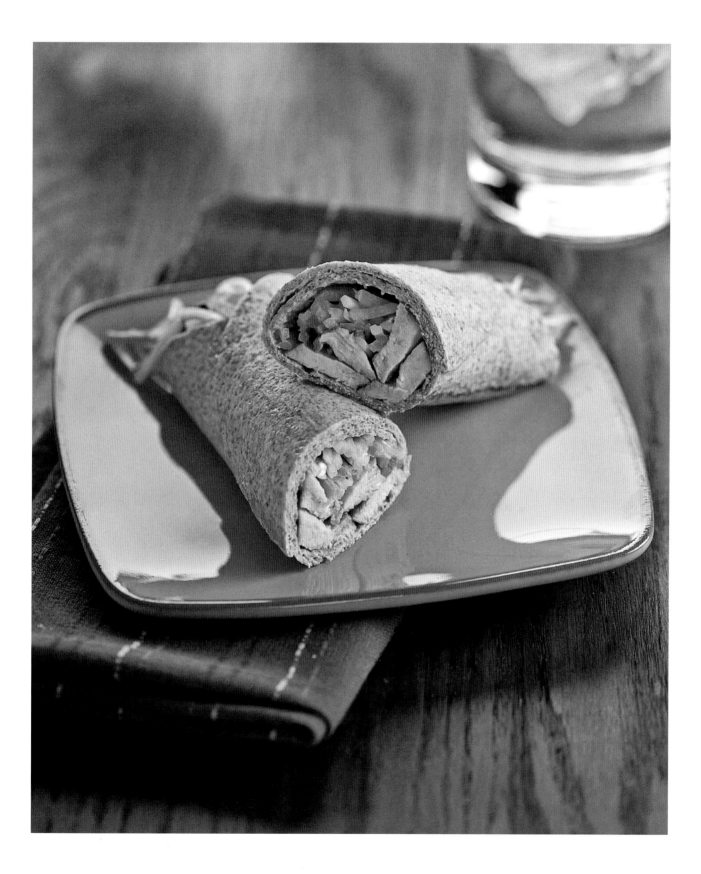

# Salmon Croquettes

1 can (14¾ ounces) pink salmon, drained and flaked

½ cup mashed potatoes*

1 egg, beaten

3 tablespoons diced red bell pepper

2 tablespoons sliced green onion

1 tablespoon chopped fresh parsley

½ cup seasoned dry bread crumbs

*Use mashed potatoes that are freshly made, leftover or ones made from instant potatoes.

1. Combine salmon, potatoes, egg, bell pepper, green onion and parsley in medium bowl; mix well.

2. Place bread crumbs on medium plate. Shape salmon mixture into 10 croquettes about 3 inches long and 1 inch wide. Roll croquettes in crumbs to coat. Refrigerate 15 to 20 minutes or until firm.

3. Preheat air fryer to 350°F. Cook in batches 6 to 8 minutes or until browned. Serve immediately.

*MAKES 5 SERVINGS*

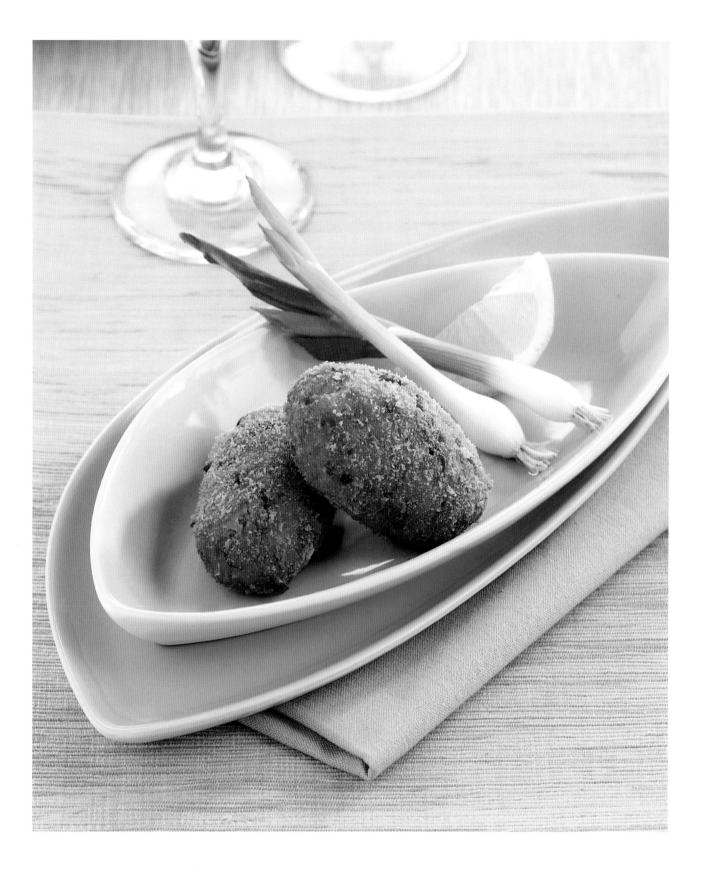

# Ricotta and Spinach Hasselback Chicken

½ cup fresh baby spinach leaves

1 teaspoon olive oil

2 tablespoons ricotta cheese

2 boneless skinless chicken breasts (about ½ to ¾ pound each)

¼ teaspoon salt

⅛ teaspoon black pepper

¼ cup (1 ounce) shredded Cheddar cheese

1. Preheat air fryer to 390°F. Line air fryer basket with foil.

2. Place spinach and oil in small microwavable dish. Microwave on HIGH 20 to 30 seconds or until spinach is slightly wilted. Stir ricotta cheese into spinach; mix well.

3. Cut four diagonal slits three fourths of the way into each chicken breast (do not cut all the way through). Place about 1 teaspoon ricotta mixture into each slit. Sprinkle chicken with salt and pepper.

4. Cook 12 minutes. Top chicken with Cheddar cheese.

5. Cook 4 to 6 minutes or until cheese is melted and chicken is golden and juices run clear.

*MAKES 2 SERVINGS*

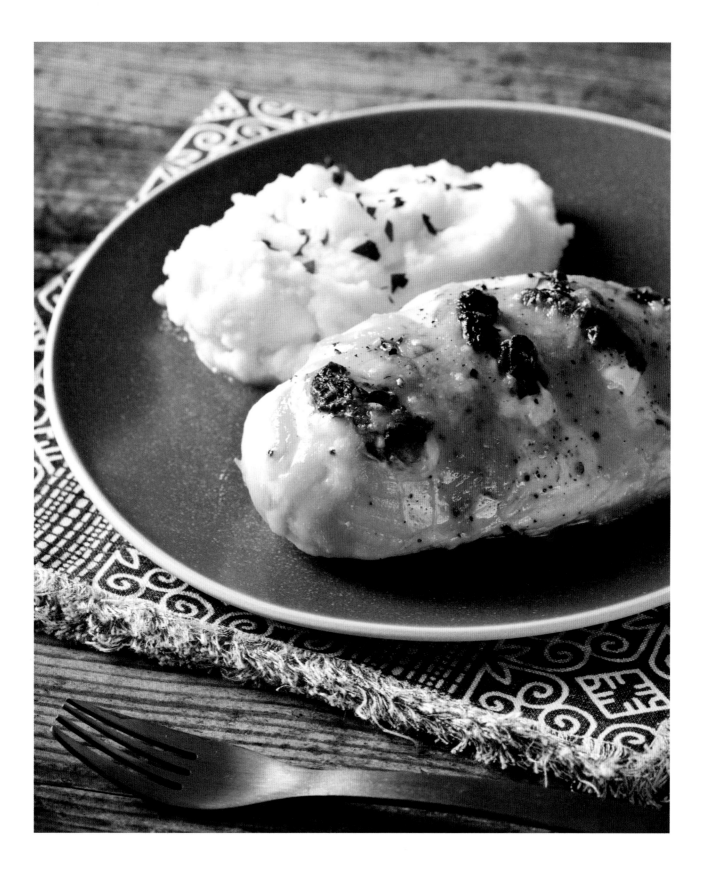

# Crispy Mustard Chicken

4  bone-in chicken breasts

Salt and black pepper

⅓  cup Dijon mustard

½  cup panko bread crumbs*
   or coarse dry bread
   crumbs

*Panko bread crumbs are used in
Japanese cooking to provide a crisp
exterior to foods. They are coarser
than ordinary bread crumbs. Panko
can be found in Asian markets or in
the Asian aisle of supermarkets.

1. Preheat air fryer to 370°F. Line air fryer basket with foil; spray with nonstick cooking spray.

2. Season chicken with salt and pepper. Cook 20 minutes.

3. Brush chicken generously with mustard. Sprinkle with panko, gently pressing panko into mustard. Cook 6 to 8 minutes or until chicken is golden brown and cooked through.

*MAKES 4 SERVINGS*

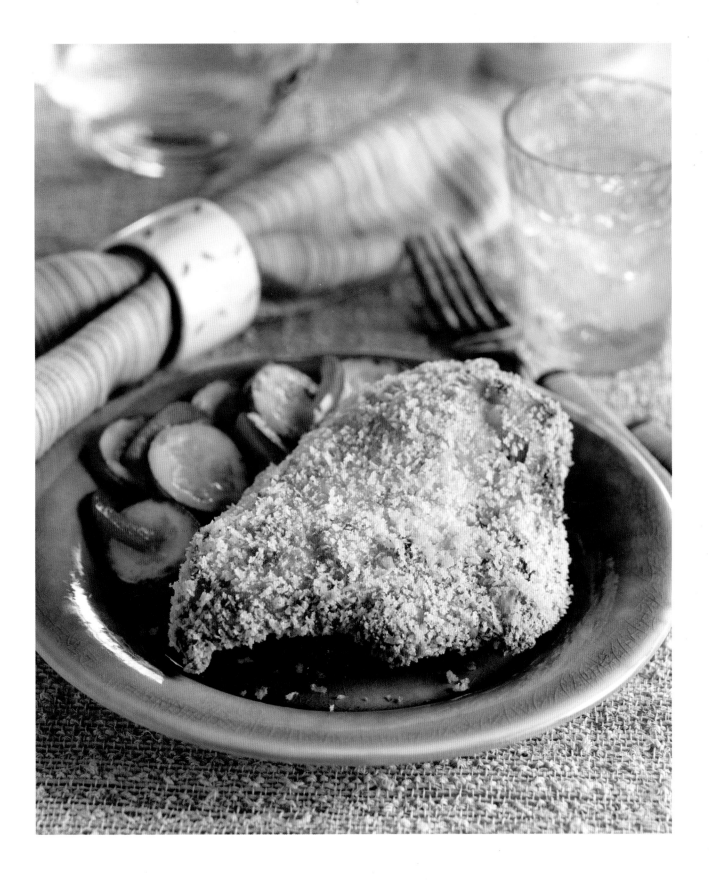

# Stuffed Party Baguette

2 medium red bell peppers

1 loaf French bread (about 14 inches long)

¼ cup plus 2 tablespoons Italian dressing, divided

1 small red onion, very thinly sliced

8 large fresh basil leaves

3 ounces Swiss cheese, very thinly sliced

1. Preheat air fryer to 390°F.

2. To roast bell peppers, cut in half; remove stems, seeds and membranes. Place peppers, cut sides down, in air fryer basket. Cook 15 minutes, turning once or twice. When done cooking, let sit in air fryer 10 minutes before removing.

3. Use paring knife to carefully remove skin. (It should easily come off.) Discard skins; cut peppers into strips.

4. Trim ends from bread. Cut loaf in half lengthwise. Remove soft insides of loaf; reserve for another use.

5. Brush ¼ cup Italian dressing evenly onto cut sides of bread. Arrange pepper strips on bottom half of loaf; top with onion. Brush onion with remaining 2 tablespoons Italian dressing; top with basil and cheese. Replace bread top. Wrap loaf tightly in plastic wrap; refrigerate at least 2 hours.

6. To serve, remove plastic wrap. Cut loaf crosswise into slices. Secure with toothpicks.

*MAKES 12 SERVINGS*

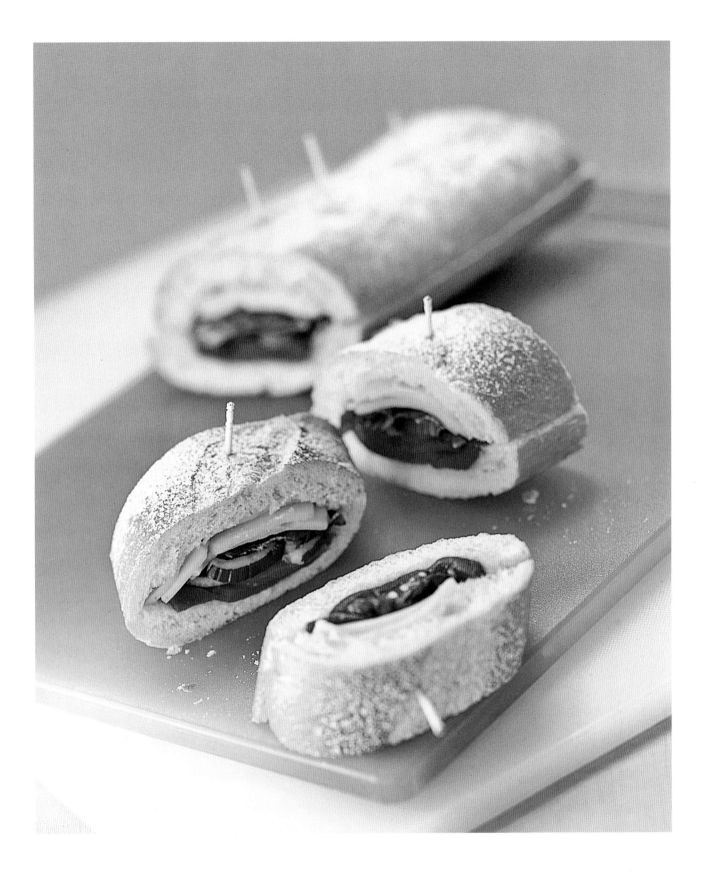

# Tuna Melts

1 can (about 5 ounces) chunk white tuna packed in water, drained and flaked

½ cup packaged coleslaw mix

1 tablespoon sliced green onion

1 tablespoon mayonnaise

½ tablespoon Dijon mustard

¼ teaspoon dried dill weed (optional)

2 English muffins, split

¼ cup (1 ounce) shredded Cheddar cheese

1. Preheat air fryer to 370°F. Combine tuna, coleslaw mix and green onion in medium bowl. Combine mayonnaise, mustard and dill weed, if desired, in small bowl. Stir mayonnaise mixture into tuna mixture. Spread tuna mixture onto muffin halves.

2. Cook 3 to 4 minutes or until heated through and lightly browned. Sprinkle with cheese. Cook 1 to 2 minutes until cheese is melted.

*MAKES 2 SERVINGS*

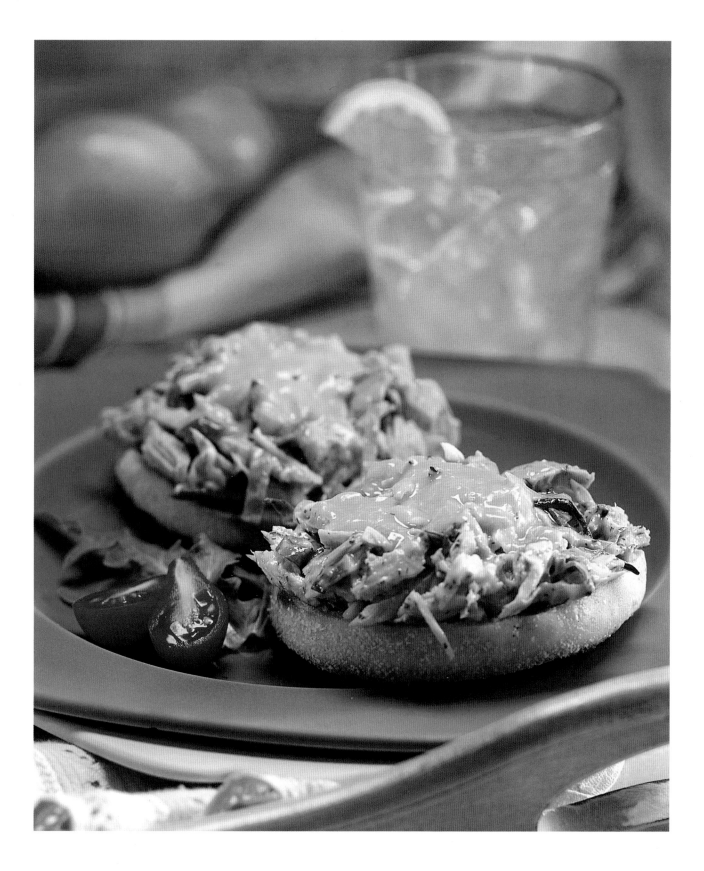

# Air-Fried Cajun Bass

2 tablespoons all-purpose flour

1 to 1½ teaspoons Cajun or Caribbean jerk seasoning

1 egg white

2 teaspoons water

⅓ cup seasoned dry bread crumbs

2 tablespoons cornmeal

4 skinless striped bass, halibut or cod fillets (4 to 6 ounces each), thawed if frozen

Chopped fresh parsley (optional)

4 lemon wedges

1. Combine flour and seasoning in medium resealable food storage bag. Whisk egg white and water in small bowl. Combine bread crumbs and cornmeal in separate small bowl.

2. Working one at a time, add fillet to bag; shake to coat evenly. Dip in egg white mixture, letting excess drip back into bowl. Roll in bread crumb mixture, pressing lightly to adhere. Repeat with remaining fillets.

3. Preheat air fryer to 390°F. Cook in batches 8 to 10 minutes, turning halfway through cooking, until golden brown and fish is opaque in center and flakes easily when tested with fork.

4. Sprinkle parsley over fish, if desired. Serve with lemon wedges.

*MAKES 4 SERVINGS*

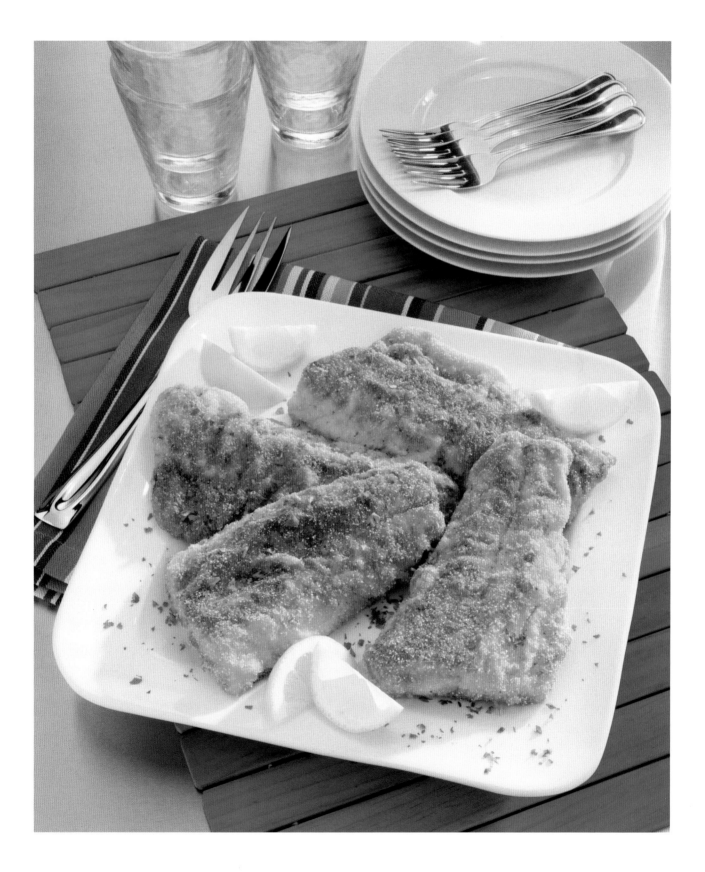

# Crispy Ranch Chicken Bites

1 pound boneless skinless
   chicken breasts

¾ cup ranch dressing, plus
   additional for serving

2 cups panko bread crumbs

1. Preheat air fryer to 370°F. Line air fryer basket with parchment paper.

2. Cut chicken into 1-inch cubes. Place ¾ cup dressing in small bowl. Spread panko in shallow dish. Dip chicken in dressing; shake off excess. Roll in panko to coat. Spray chicken with nonstick cooking spray.

3. Cook in batches 8 to 10 minutes or until golden brown and cooked through. Serve with additional ranch dressing.

*MAKES 4 SERVINGS*

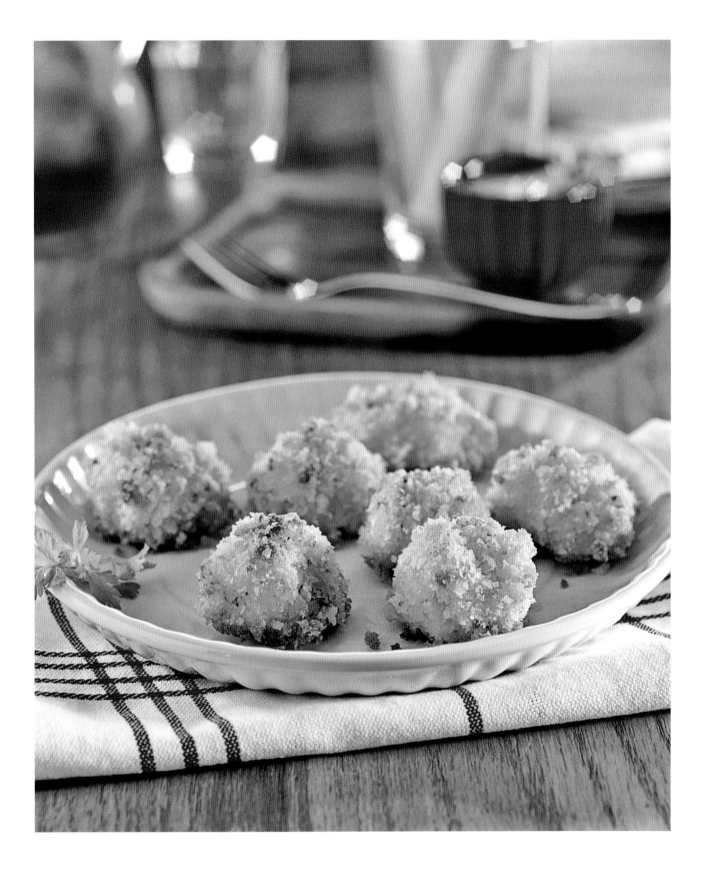

# Spicy Eggplant Burgers

1 eggplant (1¼ pounds), peeled

2 egg whites

½ cup Italian-style panko bread crumbs

3 tablespoons chipotle mayonnaise or regular mayonnaise

4 whole wheat hamburger buns, warmed

1½ cups loosely packed baby spinach

8 thin slices tomato

4 slices pepper jack cheese

1. Preheat air fryer to 370°F. Line air fryer basket with foil. Cut four ½-inch thick slices from widest part of eggplant. Beat egg whites in shallow bowl. Place panko on medium plate.

2. Dip eggplant slices in egg whites; dredge in panko, pressing gently to adhere. Spray with nonstick cooking spray.

3. Cook in batches 6 to 8 minutes on each side or until golden brown.

4. Spread mayonnaise on bottom halves of buns; top with spinach, tomatoes and eggplant slice. Top with cheese and tops of buns.

*MAKES 4 SERVINGS*

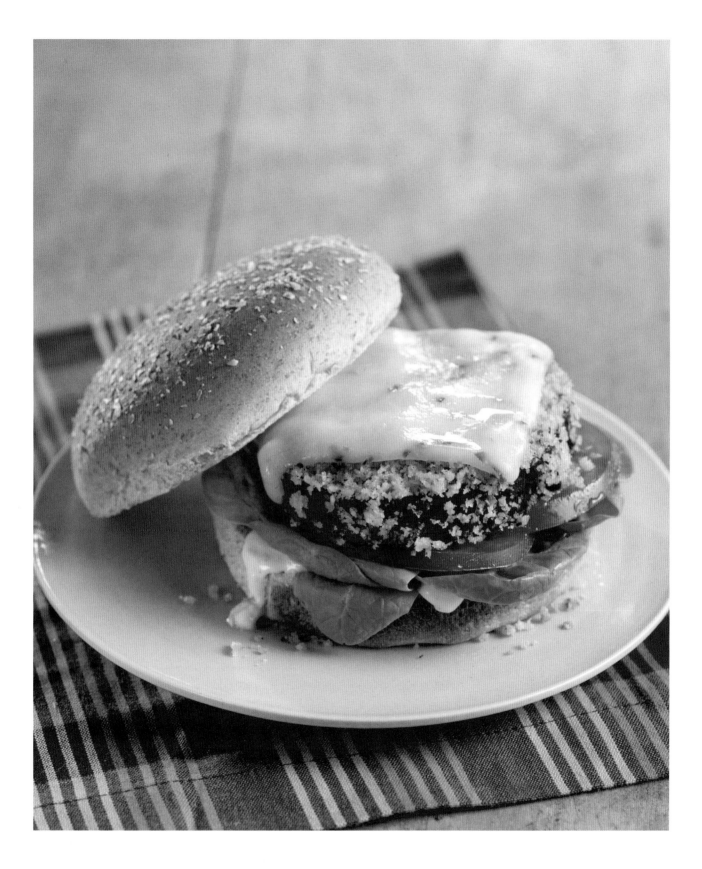

# Southern Crab Cakes with Rémoulade Dipping Sauce

10 ounces fresh lump crabmeat

1½ cups fresh white or sourdough bread crumbs, divided

¼ cup chopped green onions

½ cup mayonnaise, divided

1 egg white, lightly beaten

2 tablespoons coarse-grained or spicy brown mustard, divided

¾ teaspoon hot pepper sauce, divided

Lemon wedges (optional)

1. Pick out and discard any shell or cartilage from crabmeat. Combine crabmeat, ¾ cup bread crumbs and green onions in medium bowl. Add ¼ cup mayonnaise, egg white, 1 tablespoon mustard and ½ teaspoon hot pepper sauce; mix well. Using ¼ cup mixture per cake, shape into eight ½-inch-thick cakes. Roll crab cakes lightly in remaining ¾ cup bread crumbs.

2. Preheat air fryer to 370°F. Cook in batches 8 to 10 minutes or until golden brown, turning halfway through cooking. Transfer to serving platter; keep warm in oven.

3. For dipping sauce, combine remaining ¼ cup mayonnaise, 1 tablespoon mustard and ¼ teaspoon hot pepper sauce in small bowl; mix well.

4. Serve crab cakes with dipping sauce and lemon wedges, if desired.

*MAKES 8 SERVINGS*

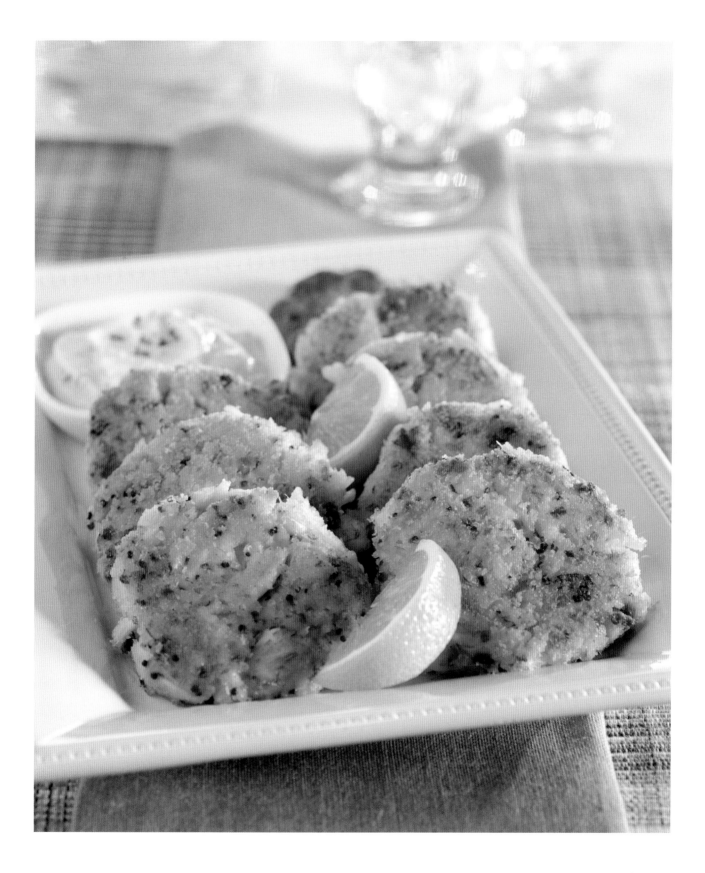

# Japanese Fried Chicken on Watercress

1 pound boneless skinless chicken breasts, cut into 2-inch pieces

3 tablespoons tamari or soy sauce

2 tablespoons sake

3 cloves garlic, minced

1 teaspoon minced fresh ginger

⅓ cup cornstarch

3 tablespoons all-purpose flour

## SALAD

¼ cup unseasoned rice vinegar

3 teaspoons tamari or soy sauce

1 teaspoon dark sesame oil

2 bunches watercress, trimmed of tough stems

1 pint grape tomatoes, halved

1. Place chicken in large resealable food storage bag. Mix 3 tablespoons tamari, sake, garlic and ginger in small bowl. Pour over chicken and marinate in refrigerator at least 30 minutes, turning bag occasionally.

2. Meanwhile, preheat air fryer to 390°F. Combine cornstarch and flour in shallow dish. Drain chicken and discard marinade. Roll chicken pieces in cornstarch mixture and shake off excess.

3. Cook in batches 8 to 10 minutes or until golden brown.

4. For salad, whisk together vinegar, 3 teaspoons tamari and sesame oil in small bowl. Arrange watercress and tomatoes on serving plates. Drizzle with dressing and top with chicken.

*MAKES 4 SERVINGS*

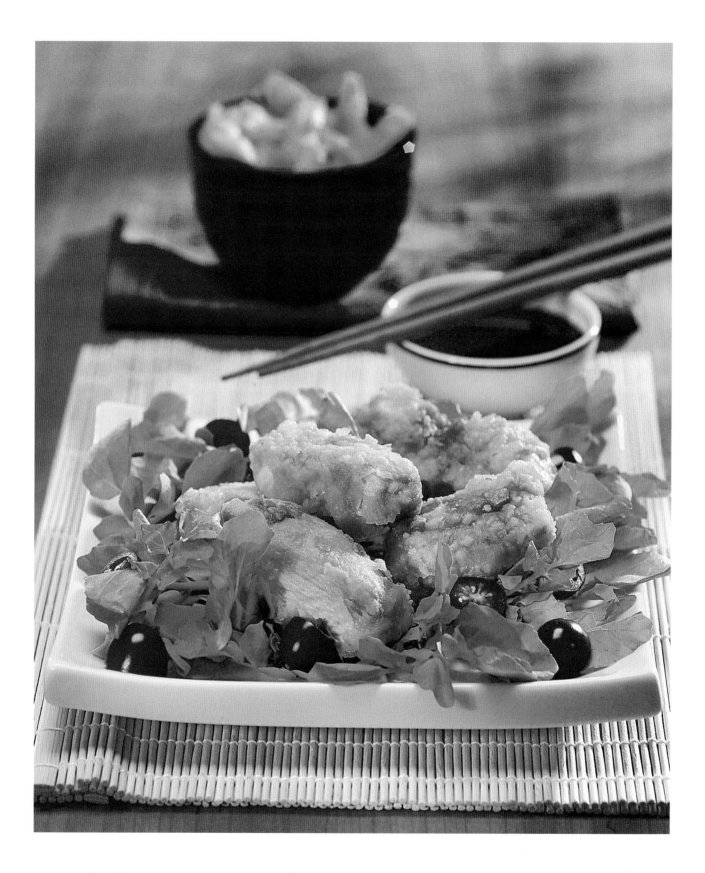

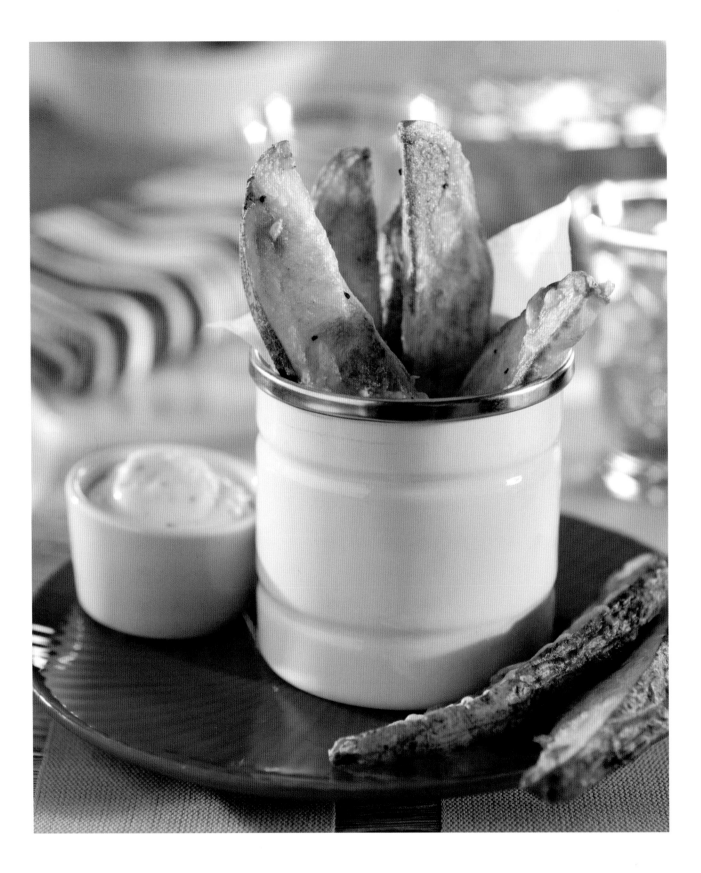

# On the Side

# Butternut Squash Fries

½ teaspoon garlic powder

¼ teaspoon salt

¼ teaspoon ground red pepper

1 butternut squash (about 2½ pounds), peeled, seeded and cut into 2-inch-thin slices

2 teaspoons vegetable oil

1. Combine garlic powder, salt and ground red pepper in small bowl; set aside.

2. Drizzle squash with oil and sprinkle with seasoning mix; gently toss to coat.

3. Preheat air fryer to 390°F. Cook in batches 16 to 18 minutes or until squash just begins to brown, shaking halfway through cooking.

*MAKES 4 SERVINGS*

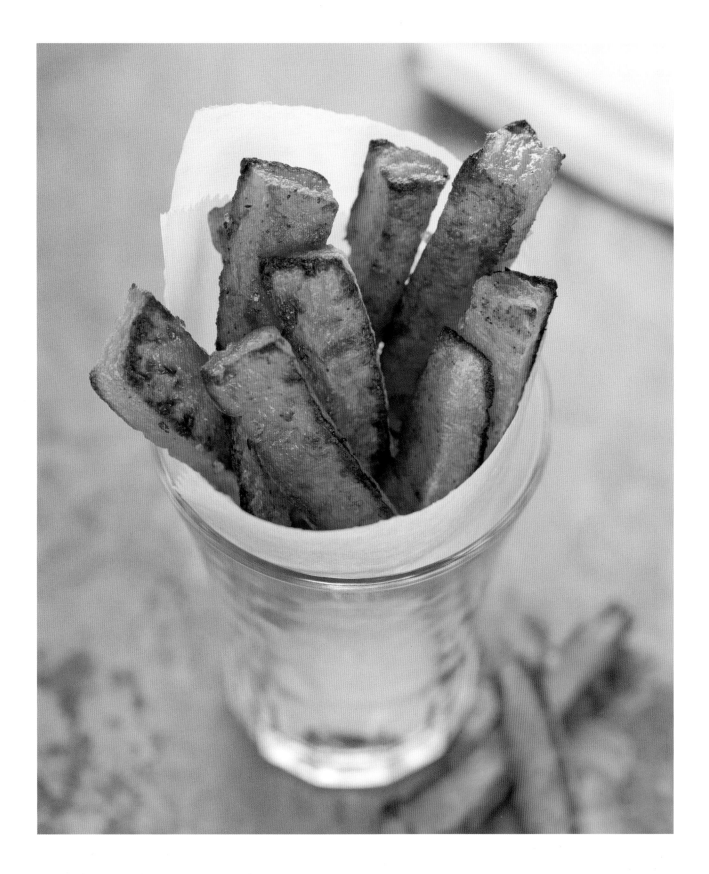

# Green Bean Fries

## DIPPING SAUCE

- ½ cup mayonnaise
- ¼ cup sour cream
- ¼ cup buttermilk
- ¼ cup minced peeled cucumber
- 1½ teaspoons lemon juice
- 1 clove garlic
- 1 teaspoon wasabi powder
- 1 teaspoon prepared horseradish
- ½ teaspoon dried dill weed
- ½ teaspoon dried parsley flakes
- ½ teaspoon salt
- ⅛ teaspoon ground red pepper

## GREEN BEAN FRIES

- 8 ounces fresh green beans, trimmed
- ½ cup all-purpose flour
- ½ cup cornstarch
- ¾ cup milk
- 1 egg
- 1 cup plain dry bread crumbs
- 1 teaspoon salt
- ½ teaspoon onion powder
- ¼ teaspoon garlic powder

1. For dipping sauce, combine mayonnaise, sour cream, buttermilk, cucumber, lemon juice, garlic, wasabi, horseradish, dill weed, parsley flakes, salt and ground red pepper in blender; blend until smooth. Refrigerate until ready to use.

2. For green bean fries, bring large saucepan of salted water to a boil. Add green beans; cook 4 minutes or until crisp-tender. Drain and run under cold running water to stop cooking.

3. Combine flour and cornstarch in large bowl. Whisk milk and egg in another large bowl. Combine bread crumbs, salt, onion powder and garlic powder in shallow bowl. Place green beans in flour mixture; toss to coat. Working in batches, coat beans with egg mixture, letting excess drain back into bowl. Roll green beans in bread crumb mixture to coat.

4. Preheat air fryer to 390°F. Cook in batches 5 to 7 minutes or until golden brown, shaking halfway through cooking. Serve warm with dipping sauce.

*MAKES 4 TO 6 SERVINGS*

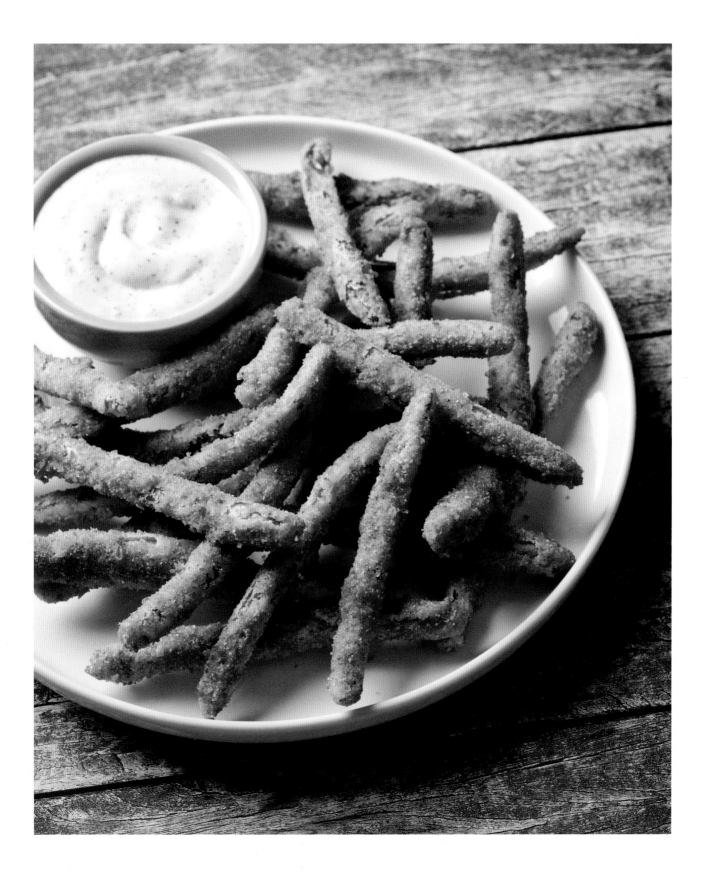

# Grilled Eggplant Roll-Ups

4 tablespoons hummus

4 slices grilled eggplant
   (recipe follows)

¼ cup crumbled feta cheese

¼ cup chopped green onions

4 tomato slices

1. Spread 1 tablespoon hummus on each eggplant slice. Top with feta, green onions and tomato.

2. Roll up tightly. Serve immediately.

*MAKES 2 SERVINGS*

**Grilled Eggplant:** Preheat air fryer to 350°F. Spray air fryer basket with nonstick cooking spray. Sprinkle four 1-inch-thick eggplant slices with ½ teaspoon salt; let stand 15 minutes. Brush eggplant with olive oil. Cook in batches 5 minutes; turn and brush with olive oil. Cook 5 minutes or until tender.

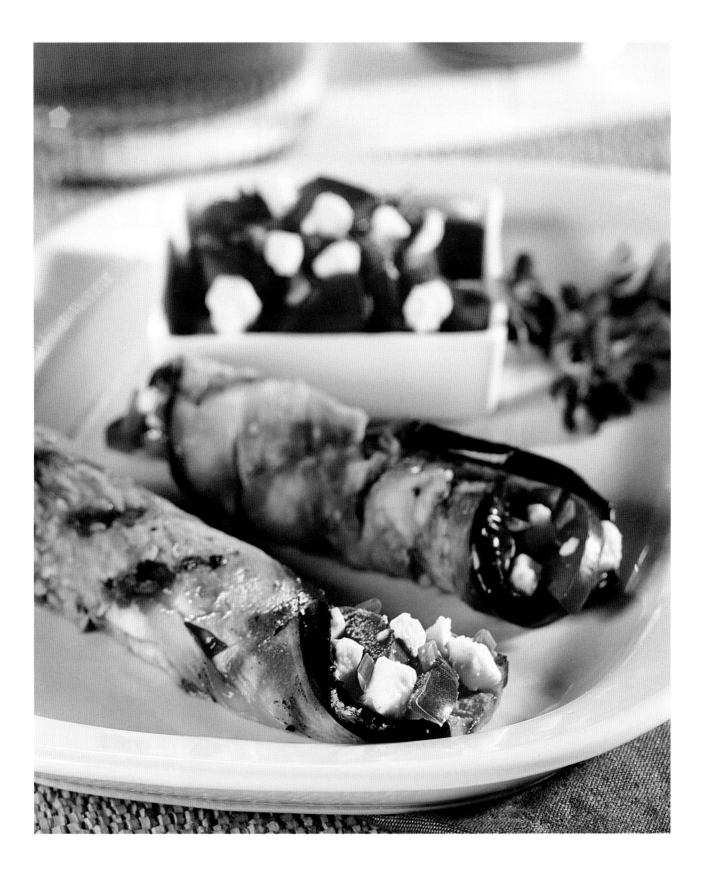

# Crispy Fries
# with Herbed Dipping Sauce

Herbed Dipping Sauce
(recipe follows)

2 large baking potatoes

2 tablespoons vegetable oil

1 teaspoon kosher salt

1. Preheat air fryer to 390°F. Spray air fryer basket with nonstick cooking spray. Prepare Herbed Dipping Sauce; set aside.

2. Cut potatoes into ¼-inch strips. Toss potato strips with oil in large bowl to coat evenly.

3. Cook in batches 18 to 20 minutes or until golden brown and crispy, shaking halfway through cooking. Sprinkle with salt. Serve immediately with Herbed Dipping Sauce.

*MAKES 3 SERVINGS*

**Herbed Dipping Sauce:** Stir ½ cup mayonnaise, 2 tablespoons chopped fresh herbs (such as basil, parsley, oregano and/or dill), 1 teaspoon salt and ½ teaspoon black pepper in small bowl until smooth and well blended. Cover and refrigerate until ready to serve.

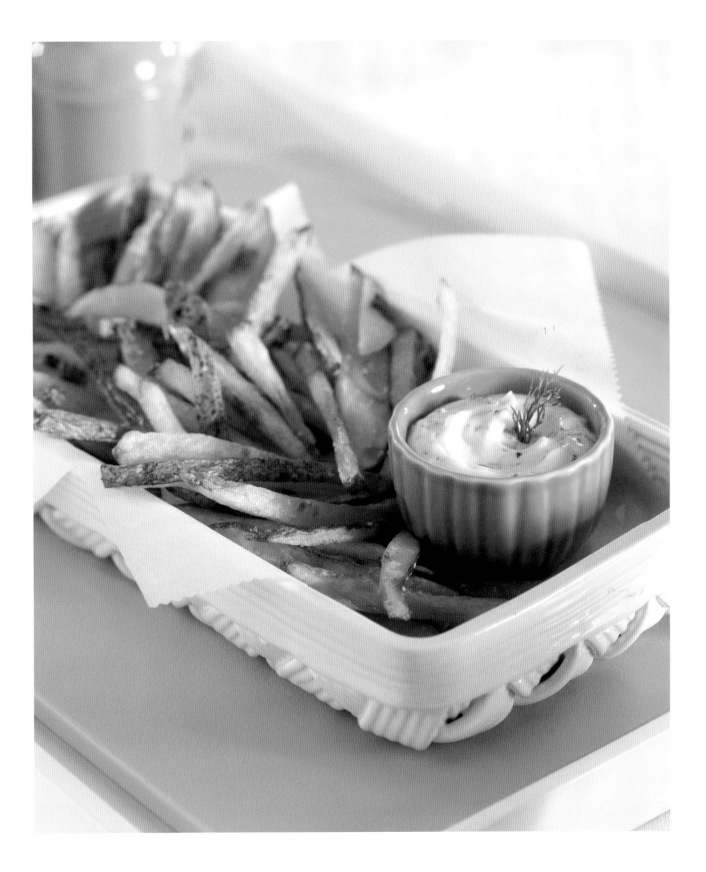

# Air-Fried Corn-on-the-Cob

2 tablespoons butter, melted

½ teaspoon salt

½ teaspoon black pepper

½ teaspoon chopped fresh parsley

2 ears corn, husks and silks removed

Foil

Grated Parmesan cheese (optional)

1. Preheat air fryer to 390°F. Combine butter, salt, pepper and parsley in small bowl. Rub corn with butter mixture. Wrap corn in foil.*

2. Cook 10 to 12 minutes, rotating midway through cooking. Sprinkle with cheese before serving, if desired.

*MAKES 2 SERVINGS*

*\*If your air fryer basket is on the smaller side, you may need to break ears of corn in half to fit.*

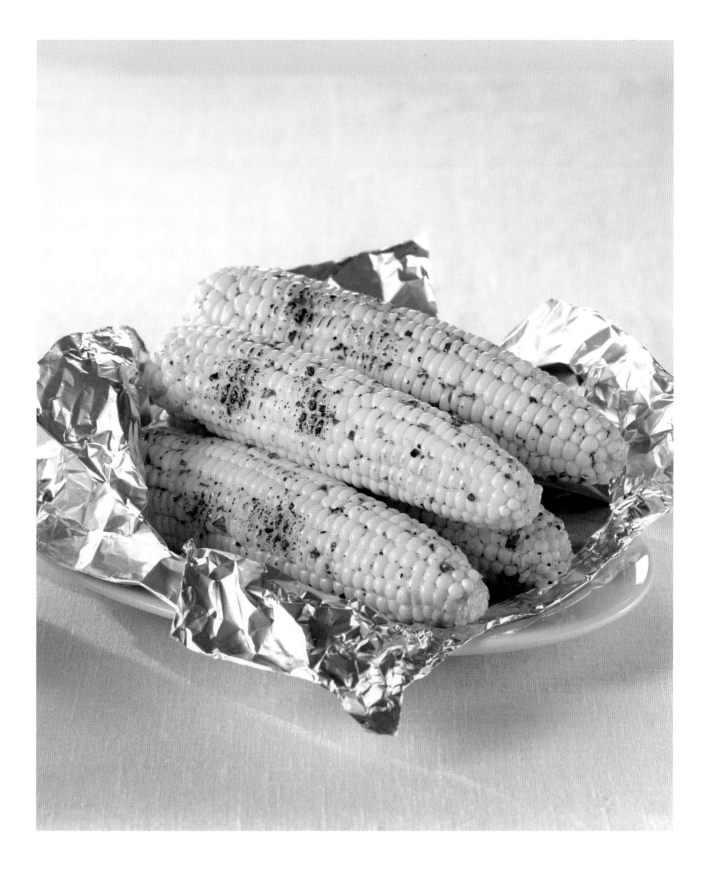

# Parmesan-Crusted French Fries with Rosemary Dipping Sauce

3 medium baking potatoes (8 ounces each), peeled and cut into 12 wedges

1 tablespoon olive oil

⅛ teaspoon salt

⅛ teaspoon black pepper

¼ cup shredded Parmesan cheese

½ cup mayonnaise

1 teaspoon chopped fresh rosemary *or* ½ teaspoon dried rosemary

½ teaspoon grated lemon peel

1 clove garlic, crushed

1. Preheat air fryer to 390°F. Toss potatoes with oil, salt and pepper in medium bowl.

2. Cook in batches 20 to 22 minutes, shaking halfway through cooking. Sprinkle cheese over potatoes. Cook additional 5 minutes or until cheese is melted and potatoes are tender.

3. Meanwhile, stir together mayonnaise, rosemary, lemon peel and garlic in small bowl. Serve potatoes with dipping sauce.

*MAKES 4 SERVINGS*

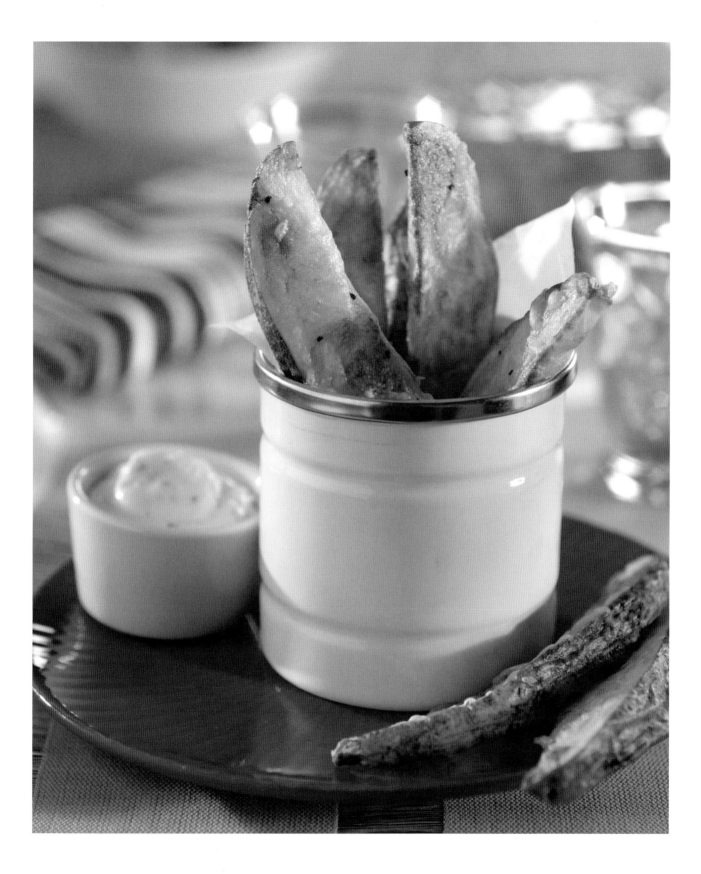

# Cheesy Garlic Bread

1 loaf (about 8 ounces) Italian bread

¼ cup (½ stick) butter, softened

4 cloves garlic, diced

2 tablespoons grated Parmesan cheese

1 cup (4 ounces) shredded mozzarella cheese

1. Preheat air fryer to 370°F. Line air fryer basket with foil.

2. Cut bread in half horizontally. Spread cut sides of bread evenly with butter; top with garlic. Sprinkle with Parmesan, then mozzarella cheeses.

3. Cook 5 to 6 minutes or until cheeses are melted and golden brown in spots. Cut crosswise into slices. Serve warm.

*MAKES 4 TO 6 SERVINGS*

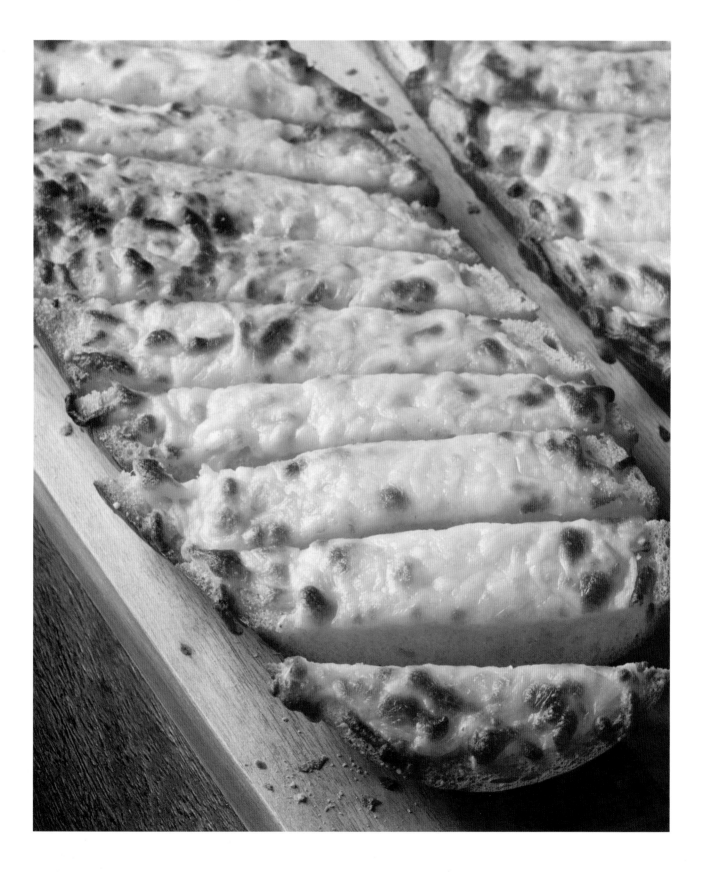

# Sweet Potato Fries

2 sweet potatoes, peeled and sliced

1 tablespoon olive oil

¼ teaspoon coarse salt

¼ teaspoon black pepper

½ cup grated Parmesan cheese (optional)

1. Preheat air fryer to 370°F. Spray air fryer basket with nonstick cooking spray.

2. Toss potatoes with oil, salt and pepper in medium bowl.

3. Cook in batches 10 to 12 minutes or until lightly browned, shaking halfway through cooking. Sprinkle with cheese, if desired.

*MAKES 2 SERVINGS*

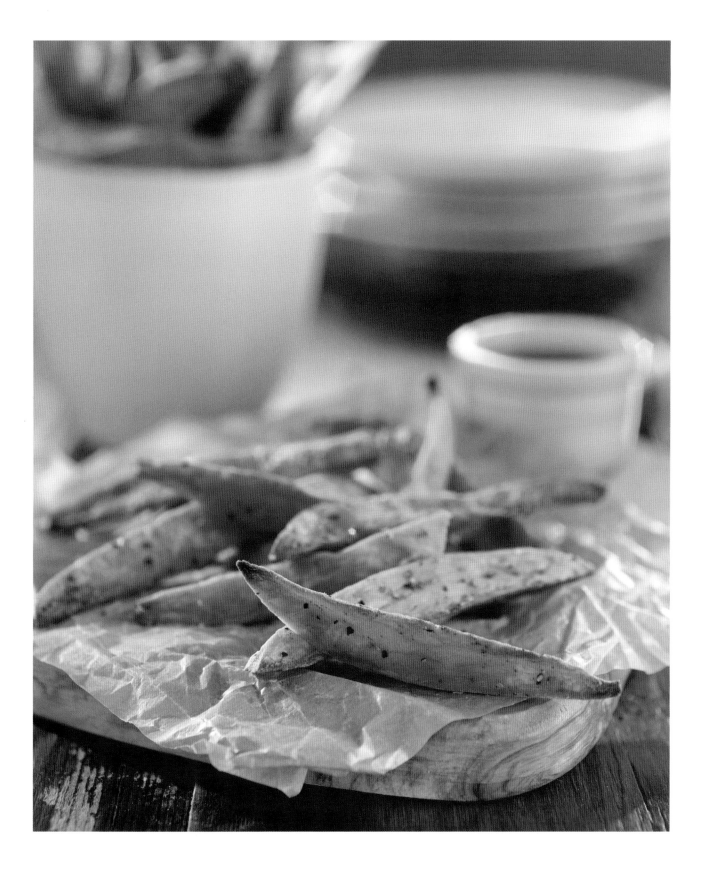

# Savory Stuffed Tomatoes

2 large ripe tomatoes
   (1 to 1¼ pounds total)

¾ cup garlic- or Caesar-
   flavored croutons

¼ cup chopped pitted
   kalamata olives (optional)

2 tablespoons chopped fresh
   basil

1 clove garlic, minced

2 tablespoons grated
   Parmesan or Romano
   cheese

1 tablespoon olive oil

1. Preheat air fryer to 350°F. Line air fryer basket with foil or parchment paper.

2. Cut tomatoes in half crosswise; discard seeds. Scrape out and reserve pulp. Set aside tomato shells.

3. Chop up tomato pulp; place in medium bowl. Add croutons, olives, if desired, basil and garlic; toss well. Spoon mixture into tomato shells. Sprinkle with cheese and drizzle oil over shells.

4. Cook 5 to 7 minutes or until heated through.

*MAKES 4 SERVINGS*

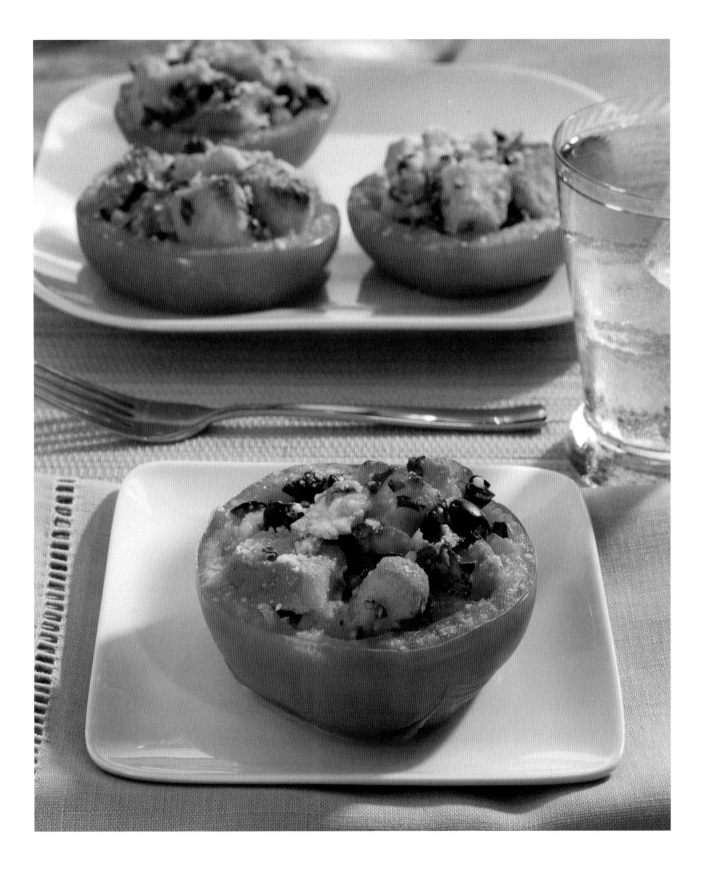

# Hasselback Potatoes

4 small Yukon Gold potatoes

3 tablespoons butter, melted and divided

½ teaspoon salt

¼ teaspoon ground black pepper

¼ cup grated Parmesan cheese

Chopped fresh parsley

1. Preheat air fryer to 390°F.

2. Cut diagonal slits into each potato about ⅛ inch apart and ¾ inches down (do not cut all the way through). Brush 2 tablespoons butter over tops; sprinkle with salt and pepper.

3. Cook 20 to 22 minutes or until slightly softened and lightly browned.

4. Brush potatoes with remaining butter. Sprinkle with cheese. Cook 3 to 5 minutes. Sprinkle with parsley.

*MAKES 4 SERVINGS*

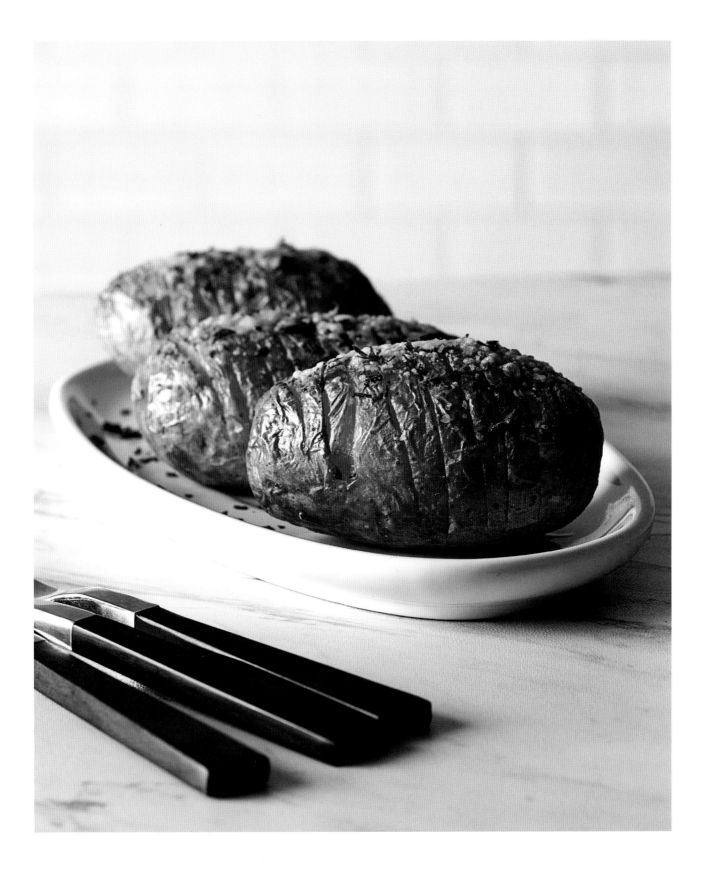

# Fried Cauliflower Florets

1 head cauliflower

1 tablespoon olive oil

½ teaspoon salt

¼ teaspoon ground black pepper

½ teaspoon chopped fresh parsley

3 tablespoons grated Parmesan cheese

2 tablespoons panko bread crumbs

1. Preheat air fryer to 370°F. Spray air fryer basket with nonstick cooking spray.

2. Cut cauliflower into florets. Place in large bowl. Drizzle with oil. Sprinkle with salt, pepper and parsley.

3. Cook in batches 6 minutes or until golden brown and slightly tender, shaking halfway through cooking.

4. Combine cheese and panko in small bowl. Sprinkle over top of cauliflower. Cook 2 to 3 minutes or until cheese has melted and golden brown.

*MAKES 2 SERVINGS*

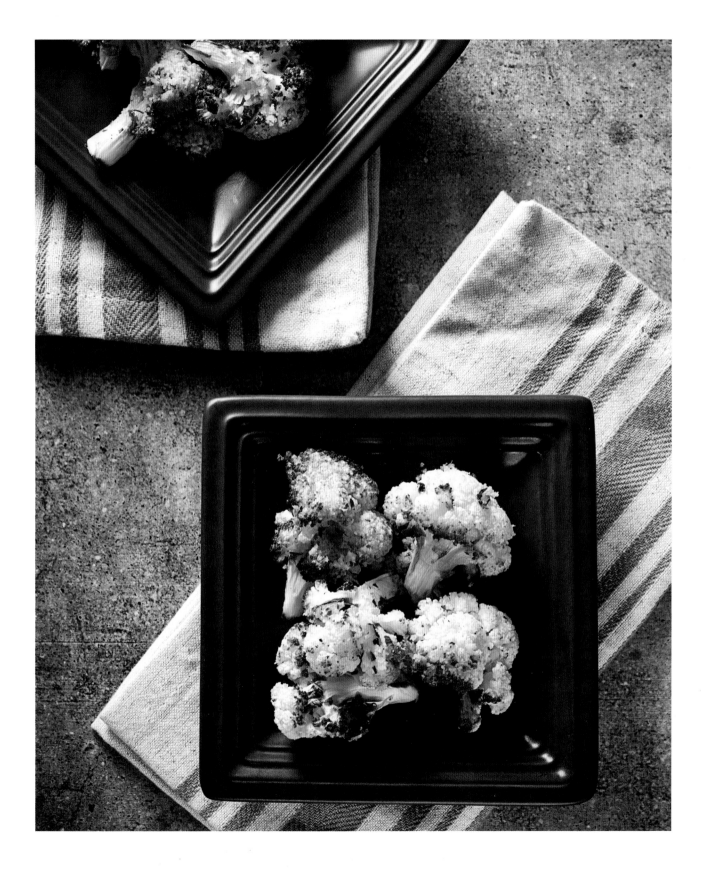

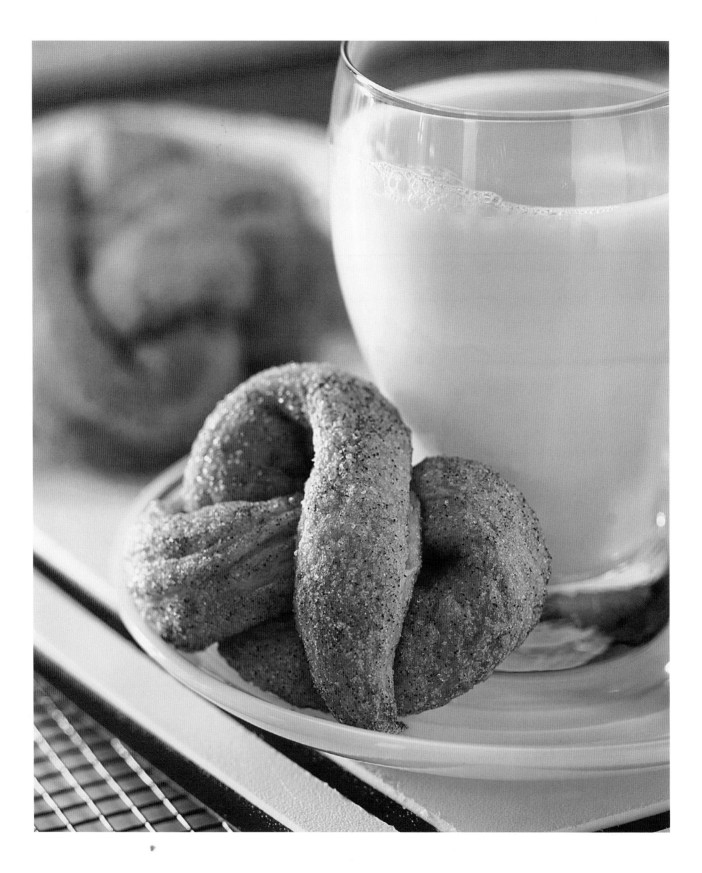

# Kids' Favorites

# Punched Pizza Rounds

1 package (12 ounces) refrigerated flaky buttermilk biscuits (10 biscuits)

80 mini pepperoni slices or 20 small pepperoni slices

1 tablespoon dried basil

½ cup pizza sauce

1½ cups (6 ounces) shredded mozzarella cheese

Shredded Parmesan cheese (optional)

1. Preheat air fryer to 370°F. Spray (2½-inch) silicone muffin cups with nonstick cooking spray.

2. Separate biscuits; split each biscuit in half horizontally to create 20 rounds. Place in prepared muffin cups. Press four mini pepperoni slices into center of each round. Sprinkle with basil. Spread pizza sauce over pepperoni; sprinkle with mozzarella.

3. Cook in batches 14 to 16 minutes or until pizzas are golden brown. Sprinkle with Parmesan, if desired. Cool 2 minutes; remove to wire racks. Serve warm.

*MAKES 20 SERVINGS*

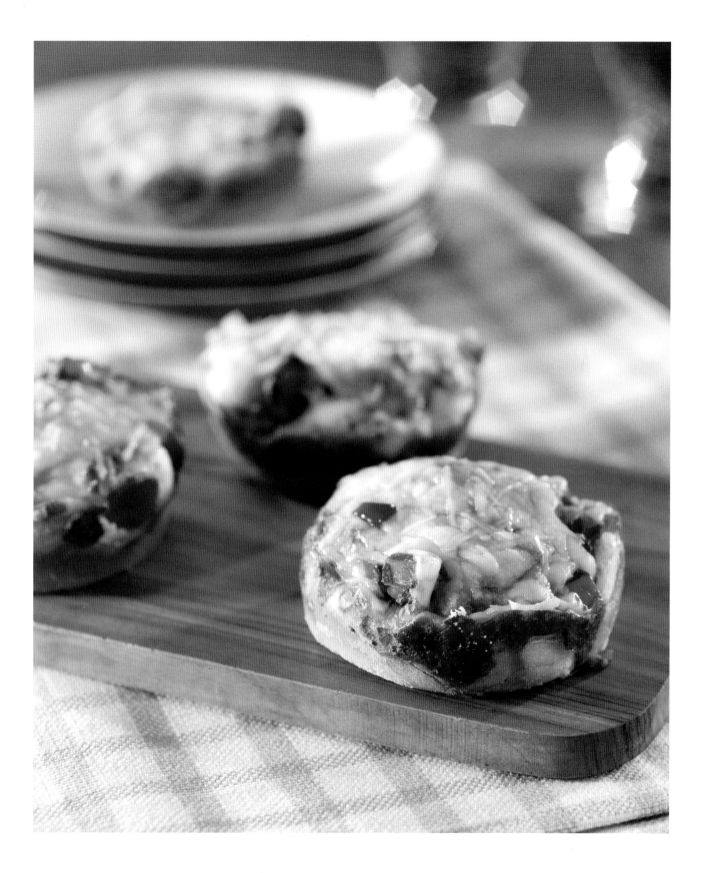

# Fried Chicken Fingers with Dipping Sauce

## DIPPING SAUCE

¼ cup plain yogurt

2 tablespoons honey

2 tablespoons prepared mustard

¼ to ½ teaspoon ground cinnamon

1 tablespoon sugar

2 teaspoons cider vinegar

⅛ teaspoon salt (optional)

⅛ teaspoon ground red pepper (optional)

## CHICKEN

1 teaspoon paprika

½ teaspoon garlic powder

½ teaspoon salt, divided

¼ teaspoon black pepper

1½ cups panko bread crumbs

⅓ cup buttermilk

2 egg whites

8 chicken tenders (about 1¼ pounds)

1. Combine Dipping Sauce ingredients in small bowl; set aside.

2. Combine paprika, garlic powder, ¼ teaspoon salt and black pepper in small bowl; set aside. Place panko in shallow dish. Whisk buttermilk and egg whites in medium bowl. Add chicken; toss until well coated.

3. Coat chicken with panko, one piece at a time, pressing down lightly to adhere. Sprinkle chicken evenly with paprika mixture.

4. Preheat air fryer to 390°F. Cook 10 to 12 minutes or until chicken is golden brown and crispy and no longer pink in center.

5. Sprinkle chicken with remaining ¼ teaspoon salt, if desired. Serve with sauce.

*MAKES 4 SERVINGS*

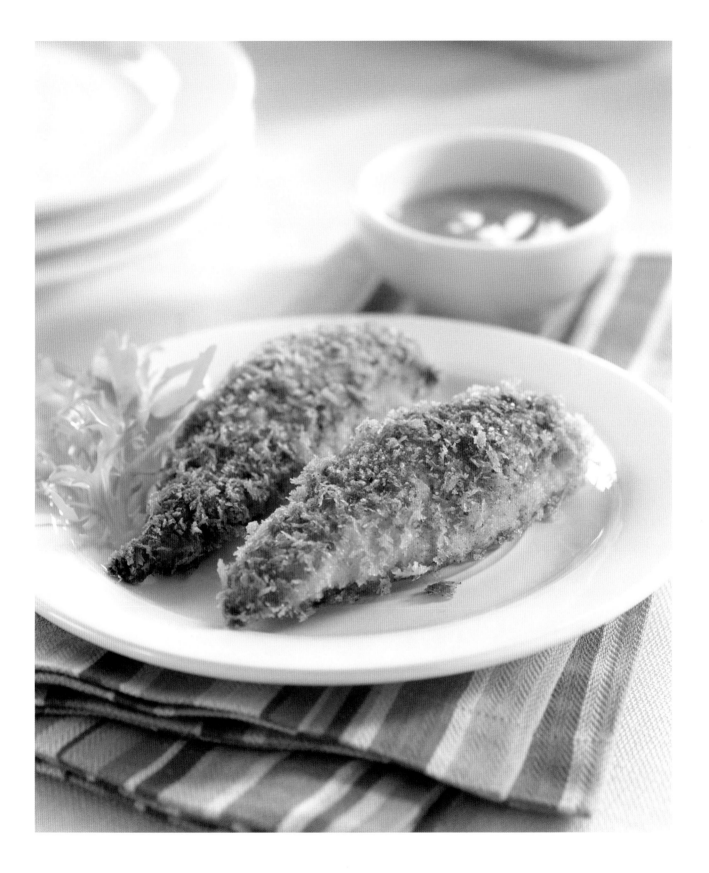

# Air-Fried S'mores

2 whole graham crackers,
   broken in half

   Foil

2 marshmallows

1 package (1.5 ounces) milk
   chocolate candy bar,
   broken in half

1. Preheat air fryer to 370°F. Prepare two s'mores at a time by placing two graham cracker squares on two sheets of foil. Top each with marshmallow. Gather foil around graham cracker.

2. Place foil packets in air fryer basket. Cook 1½ to 2 minutes or until marshmallows are browned.

3. Remove carefully from air fryer basket. Top each marshmallow with chocolate bar. Put sides together to create s'more sandwich.

*MAKES 2 SERVINGS*

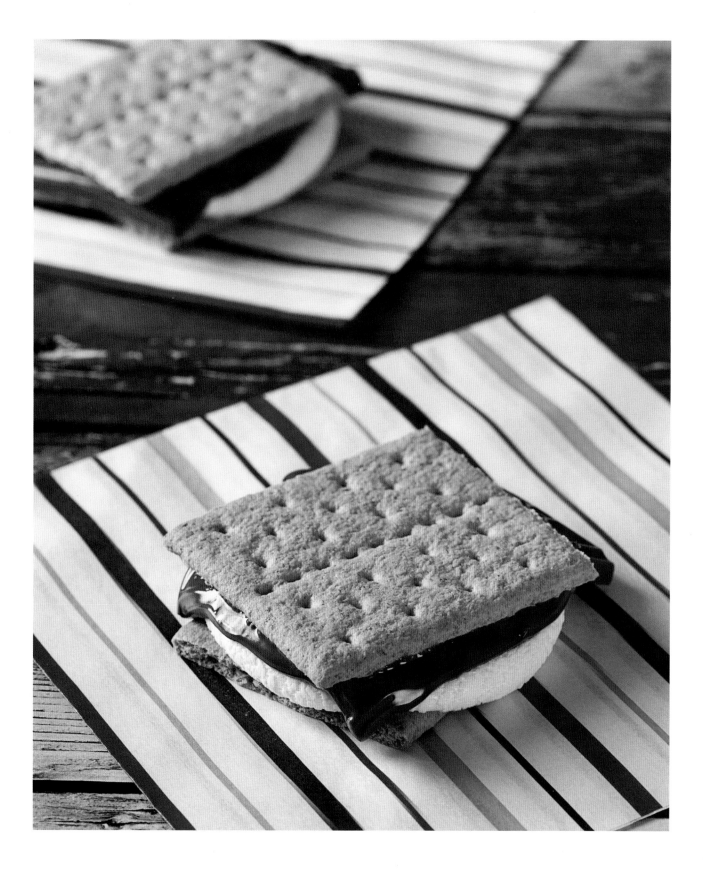

# Grilled 3-Cheese Sandwiches

2 slices (1 ounce each) Muenster cheese

2 slices (1 ounce each) Swiss cheese

2 slices (1 ounce each) Cheddar cheese

4 slices sourdough bread

2 teaspoons Dijon mustard or Dijon mustard mayonnaise

2 teaspoons melted butter

1. Preheat air fryer to 370°F.

2. Place 1 slice of each cheese on two bread slices. Spread mustard over cheese; top with remaining bread slices. Brush outsides of sandwiches with butter.

3. Cook 3 to 5 minutes or until cheeses are melted and sandwiches are golden brown.

*MAKES 2 SANDWICHES*

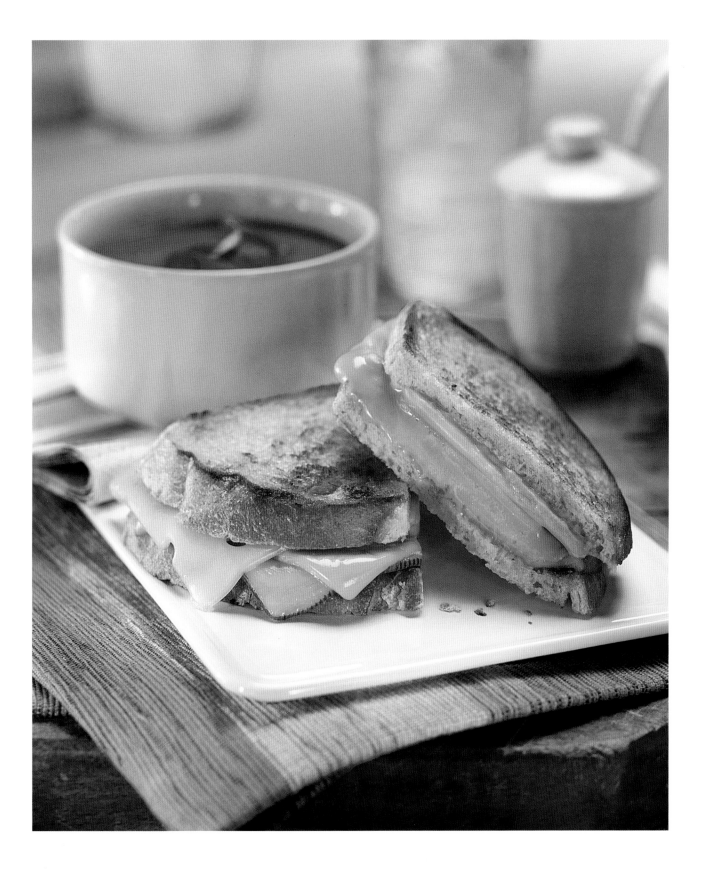

# Elephant Ears

1 sheet frozen puff pastry
   (half of 17¼-ounce
   package), thawed

1 egg, beaten

2 tablespoons sugar, divided

1 square (1 ounce) semisweet
   chocolate

1. Preheat air fryer to 370°F. Roll pastry to 12×10-inch rectangle. Brush with egg; sprinkle with 1 tablespoon sugar. Tightly roll up 10-inch sides, meeting in center. Brush center with egg and seal rolls tightly together; turn over. Cut into ⅜-inch-thick slices. Repeat with remaining pastry, egg and sugar.

2. Cook in batches 8 to 10 minutes or until golden brown. Remove to wire racks; cool completely.

3. Melt chocolate in small saucepan over low heat, stirring constantly. Remove from heat. Spread bottoms of cookies with chocolate. Place on wire rack, chocolate side up. Let stand until chocolate is set. Store between layers of waxed paper in airtight containers.

*MAKES ABOUT 2 DOZEN COOKIES*

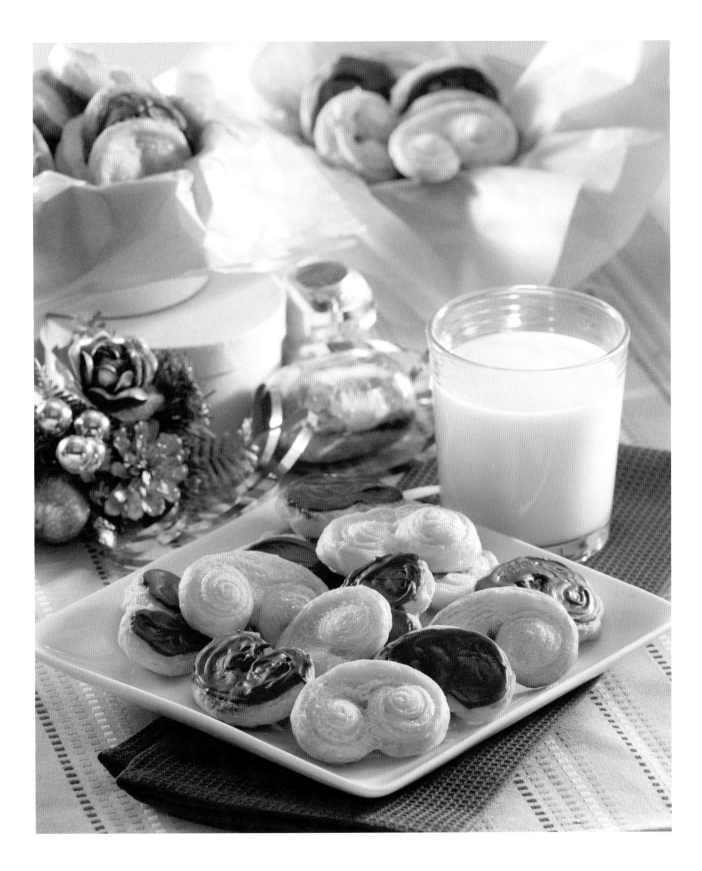

# Super Salami Twists

1 egg

1 tablespoon milk

1 cup (about ¼ pound) finely chopped hard salami

2 tablespoons yellow cornmeal

1 teaspoon Italian seasoning

1 package (about 11 ounces) refrigerated breadstick dough (12 breadsticks)

¾ cup pasta sauce, heated

1. Preheat air fryer to 350°F. Line air fryer basket with parchment paper.

2. Beat egg and milk in shallow dish until well blended. Combine salami, cornmeal and Italian seasoning in separate shallow dish.

3. Unroll breadstick dough. Separate into 12 pieces along perforations. Roll each piece of dough in egg mixture, then in salami mixture, gently pressing salami into dough. Twist each piece of dough twice.

4. Cook in batches 8 to 10 minutes or until golden brown. Remove to wire rack; cool 5 minutes. Serve warm with pasta sauce for dipping.

*MAKES 12 SERVINGS*

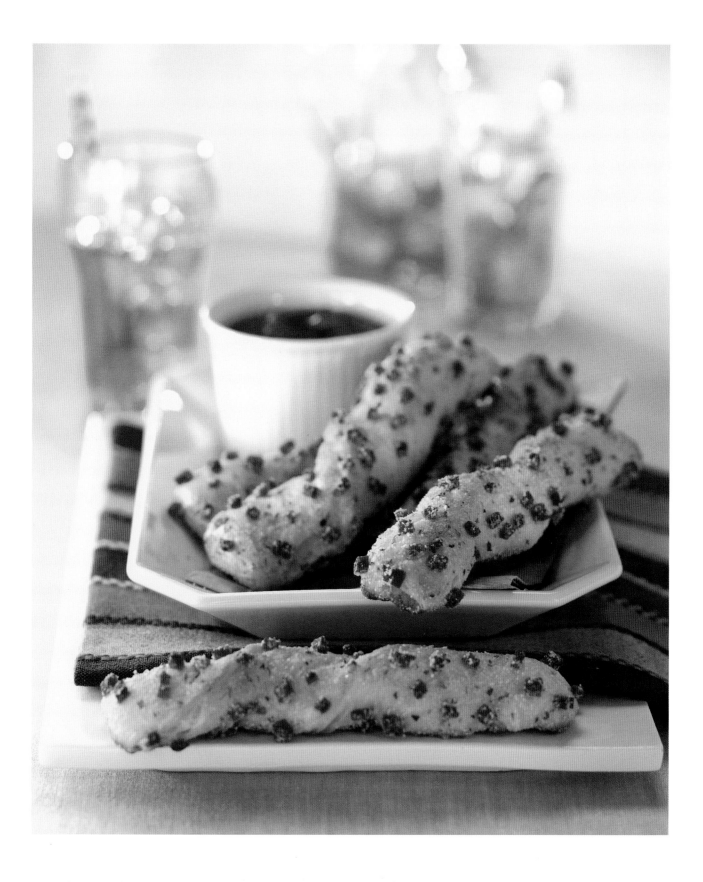

# Sugar-and-Spice Twists

2 tablespoons granulated
sugar

½ teaspoon ground cinnamon

1 package (about 11 ounces)
refrigerated breadstick
dough (12 breadsticks)

1. Preheat air fryer to 350°F. Line air fryer basket with parchment paper; spray with nonstick cooking spray.

2. Combine granulated sugar and cinnamon in shallow dish or plate. Separate breadsticks; roll each piece into 12-inch rope. Roll ropes in sugar-cinnamon mixture to coat. Twist each rope into pretzel shape.

3. Cook in batches 8 to 10 minutes or until lightly browned. Remove to wire rack to cool 5 minutes. Serve warm.

*MAKES 12 SERVINGS*

Hint: Use colored sugar sprinkles in place of the granulated sugar in this recipe for a fun "twist" of color perfect for holidays, birthdays or simple everyday celebrations.

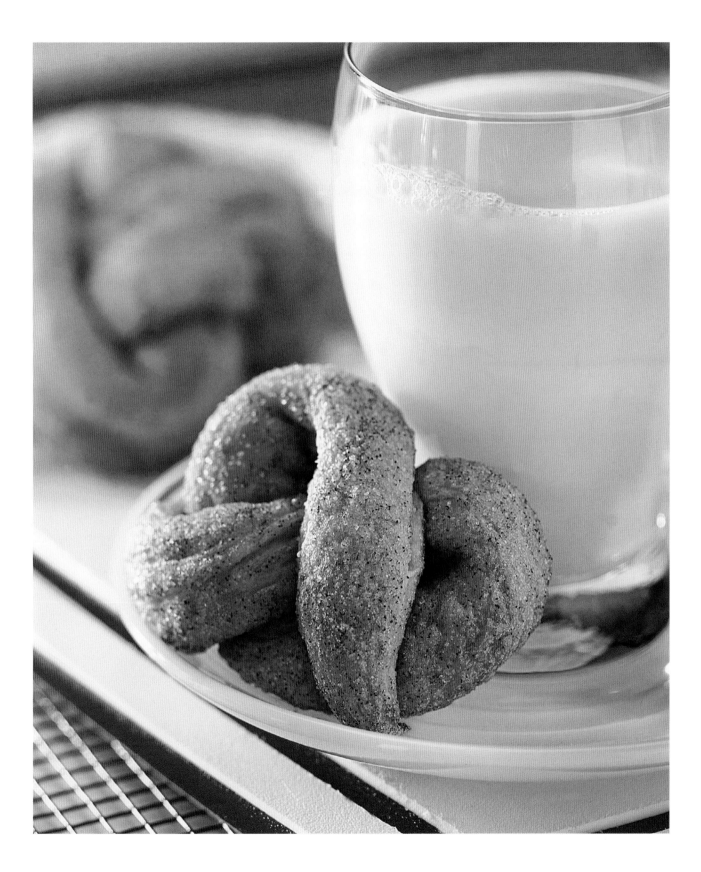

# Piggies in a Basket

1 can (8 ounces) refrigerated crescent rolls

1 package (about 12 ounces) cocktail franks

1. Preheat air fryer to 350°F.

2. Cut crescent dough into strips. Wrap dough around each frank.

3. Cook in batches 3 to 4 minutes or until golden brown.

*MAKES 4 SERVINGS*

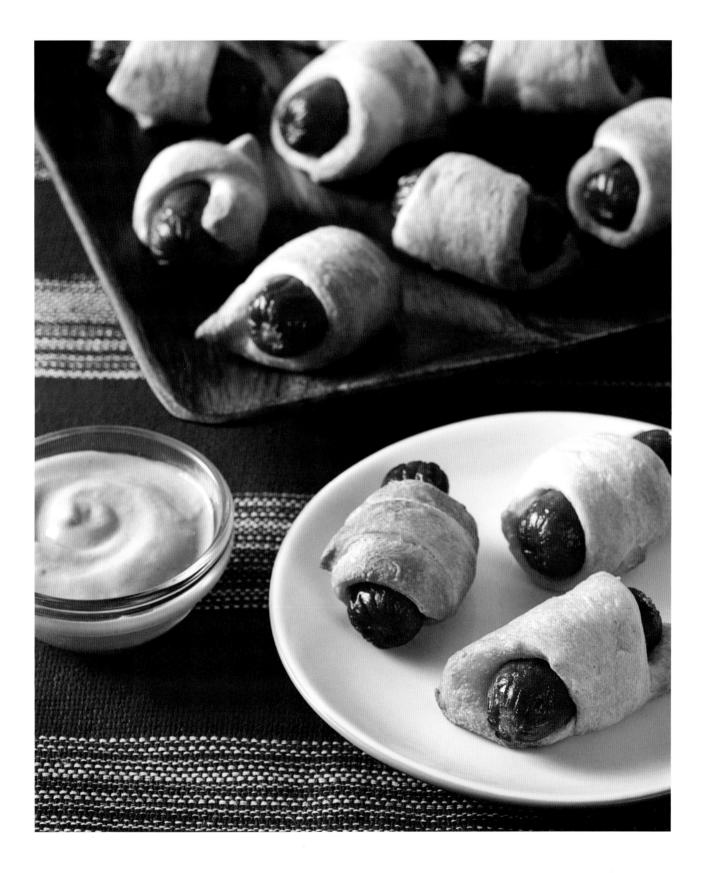

# Chocolate Rolls

½ cup sugar, divided

1 package (15 ounces) refrigerated pie crusts (2 crusts)

1 cup semisweet chocolate chips

1 egg white

Powdered sugar (optional)

1. Preheat air fryer to 370°F. Spray air fryer basket with nonstick cooking spray.

2. Sprinkle 2 tablespoons sugar on cutting board or work surface. Unroll one pie crust over sugar. Sprinkle pie crust with 2 tablespoons sugar. Using pizza wheel or sharp knife, trim away 1 inch dough from four sides to form square. (Save dough trimmings for another use or discard.)

3. Cut square in half; cut each half crosswise into four pieces to form eight 4×2-inch rectangles. Place heaping teaspoon chocolate chips at one short end of each rectangle; roll up, enclosing chocolate chips. Brush lightly with egg white. Repeat with remaining crust.

4. Cook in batches 8 to 10 minutes or until lightly browned. Cool 10 minutes to serve warm, or cool completely. Sprinkle with powdered sugar, if desired.

*MAKES 16 ROLLS*

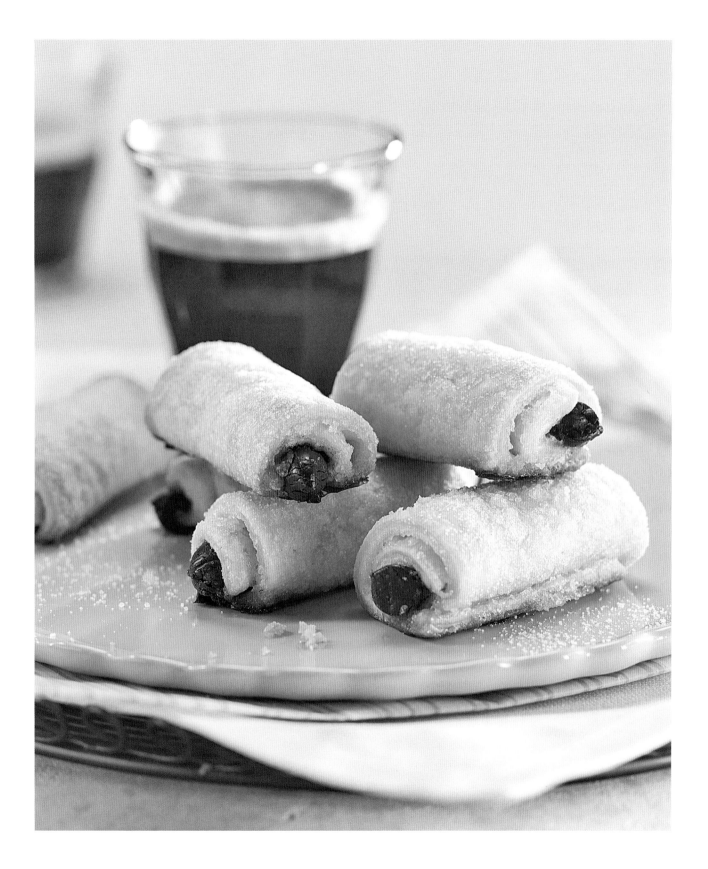

# Individual Apple Pies

1 package (15 ounces)
   refrigerated pie crusts
   (2 crusts)

   All-purpose flour

1 can (21 ounces) apple pie
   filling

3 tablespoons butter, melted

   Powdered sugar

1. Preheat air fryer to 370°F. Let crusts stand at room temperature 15 minutes. Spray air fryer basket with nonstick cooking spray.

2. Roll out each crust into 12½-inch circle on floured surface; cut out seven 4-inch circles. Place generous tablespoon of apple pie filling on half of dough circle, leaving ¼-inch border. Dip finger in water and moisten edge of one dough circle. Fold dough over filling, pressing lightly. Dip fork in flour and crimp edge of dough to seal completely. Brush butter over top.

3. Cook in batches 5 to 7 minutes or until lightly browned. Transfer pies to serving platter.

4. Sprinkle with powdered sugar; serve warm or at room temperature.

*MAKES 14 SERVINGS*

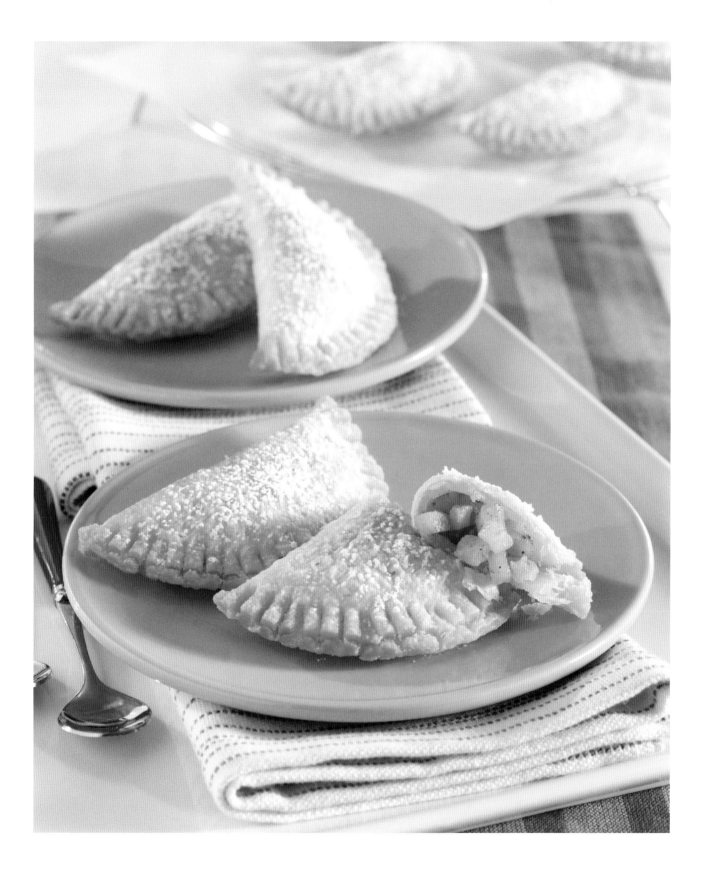

# Grilled Cheese Kabobs

8 thick slices whole wheat bread

3 thick slices sharp Cheddar cheese

3 thick slices Monterey Jack or Colby Jack cheese

2 tablespoons butter, melted

1. Cut each slice bread into 1-inch squares. Cut each slice cheese into 1-inch squares. Make small sandwiches with one square of bread and one square of each type of cheese. Top with second square of bread. Brush sandwiches with butter.

2. Preheat air fryer to 370°F. Cook sandwich squares 30 seconds to 1 minute on each side or until golden and cheese is slightly melted.

3. Place sandwiches on the ends of short wooden skewers, if desired, or eat as finger food.

*MAKES 12 SERVINGS*

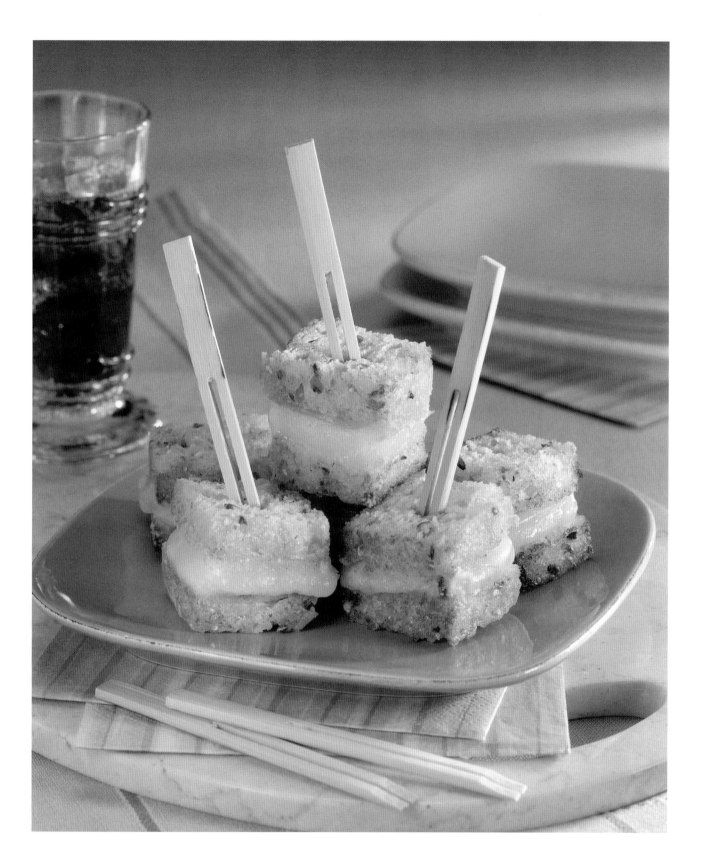

# Veggie Pizza Pitas

1 whole wheat pita bread round, cut in half horizontally (to make 2 rounds)

2 tablespoons pizza sauce

½ teaspoon dried basil

⅛ teaspoon red pepper flakes (optional)

½ cup sliced mushrooms

¼ cup thinly sliced green bell pepper

¼ cup thinly sliced red onion

½ cup (4 ounces) shredded mozzarella cheese

1 teaspoon grated Parmesan cheese

1. Preheat air fryer to 370°F.

2. Arrange pita rounds, rough sides up, in single layer. Spread 1 tablespoon pizza sauce evenly over each round to within ¼ inch of edge. Sprinkle with basil and red pepper flakes, if desired. Top with mushrooms, bell pepper and onion. Sprinkle with mozzarella cheese.

3. Cook one at a time 5 to 7 minutes or until mozzarella cheese is melted. Sprinkle ½ teaspoon Parmesan cheese over each round.

*MAKES 2 SERVINGS*

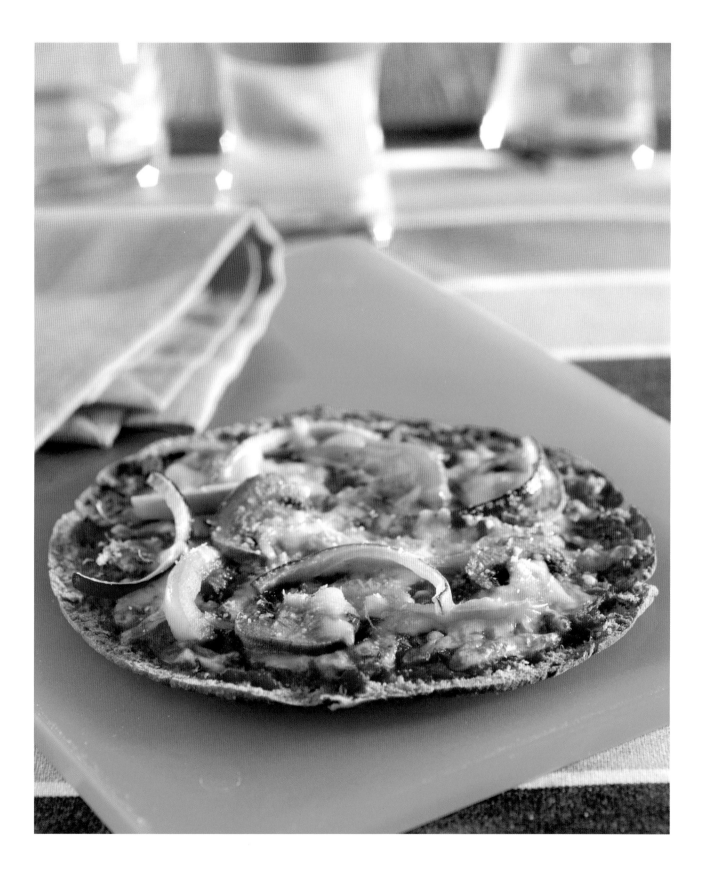

# Candy Calzone

1 package small chocolate,
  peanut and nougat candy
  bars, chocolate peanut
  butter cups or other
  chocolate candy bar
  (8 bars)

1 package (15 ounces)
  refrigerated pie crusts
  (2 crusts)

½ cup milk chocolate chips

1. Preheat air fryer to 350°F. Line air fryer basket with parchment paper. Chop candy into ¼-inch pieces.

2. Unroll pie crusts on cutting board or clean surface. Cut out 3-inch circles with biscuit cutter. Place about 1 tablespoon chopped candy on one side of each circle; fold dough over candy to form semicircle. Crimp edges with fingers or fork to seal.

3. Cook in batches 8 to 10 minutes or until golden brown. Remove to wire rack to cool slightly.

4. Place chocolate chips in small microwavable bowl; microwave on HIGH 1 minute. Stir; microwave in 30-second intervals, stirring in between, until smooth. Drizzle melted chocolate over calzones; serve warm.

*MAKES 16 SERVINGS*

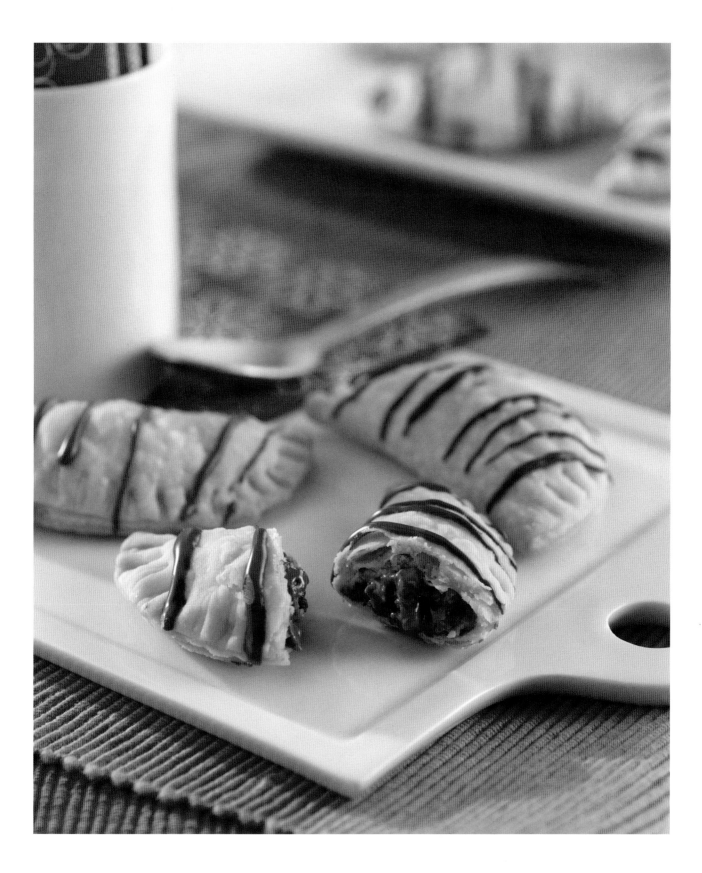

# Cinnamon Toast Poppers

6 cups fresh bread* cubes
   (1-inch cubes)

2 tablespoons butter,
   melted

1 tablespoon plus
   1½ teaspoons sugar

½ teaspoon ground cinnamon

   *Use a firm sourdough, whole wheat
   or semolina bread.

1. Preheat air fryer to 330°F. Place bread cubes in large bowl. Drizzle with butter; toss to coat.

2. Combine sugar and cinnamon in small bowl. Sprinkle over bread cubes; mix well.

3. Cook 12 to 15 minutes or until bread is golden and fragrant, shaking once or twice. Serve warm or at room temperature.

MAKES 12 SERVINGS

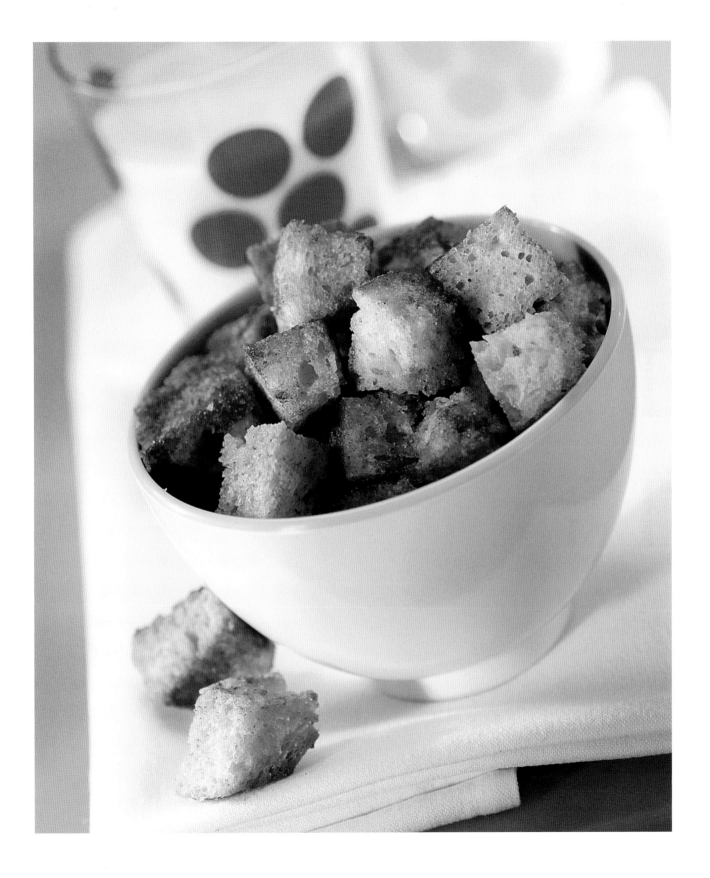

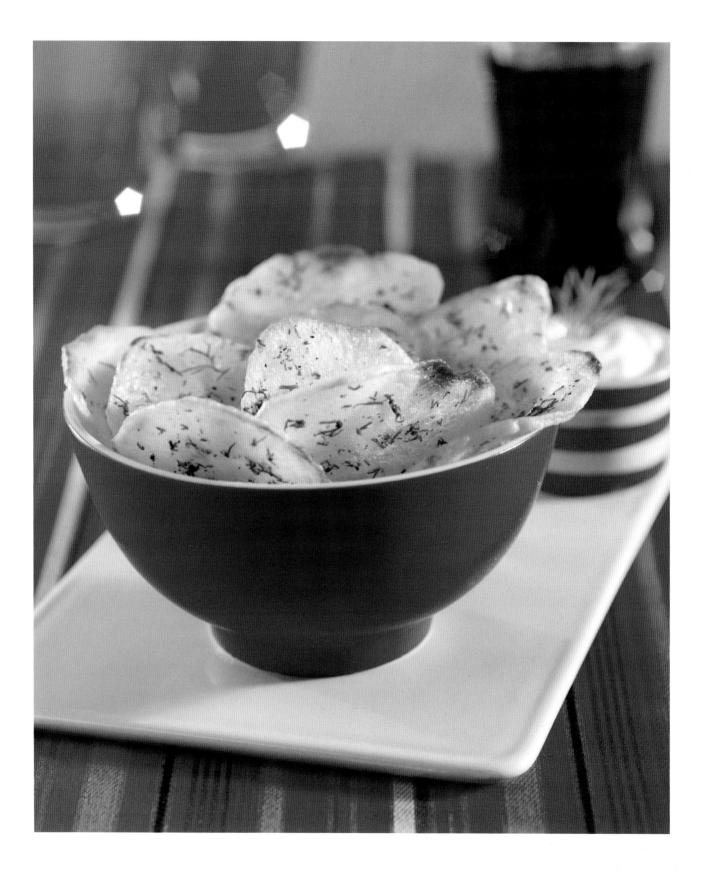

# Snacks & Chips

# Roasted Chickpeas

1 can (about 14 ounces) chickpeas, rinsed and drained

2 tablespoons olive oil

½ teaspoon salt

½ teaspoon black pepper

½ tablespoon chili powder

¼ teaspoon ground red pepper

1 lime, cut into wedges

1. Preheat air fryer to 390°F.

2. Combine chickpeas, oil, salt and black pepper in large bowl. Place in air fryer basket.

3. Cook 8 to 10 minutes or until chickpeas begin to brown, shaking pan twice.

4. Sprinkle with chili powder and ground red pepper. Serve with lime wedges.

*MAKES 1 CUP*

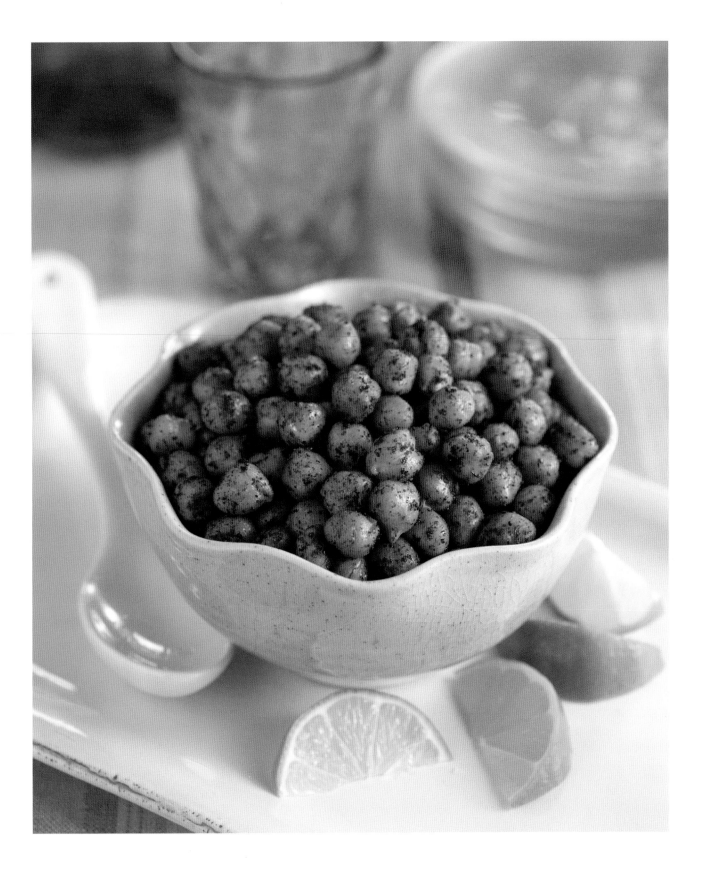

# Kale Chips

1 large bunch kale (about 1 pound)

1 to 2 tablespoons olive oil

1 teaspoon garlic powder

½ teaspoon salt

½ teaspoon black pepper

1. Preheat air fryer to 390°F.

2. Wash kale and pat dry with paper towels. Remove center ribs and stems; discard. Cut leaves into 2- to 3-inch-wide pieces.

3. Combine leaves, oil, garlic powder, salt and pepper in large bowl; toss to coat.

4. Cook in batches 3 to 4 minutes or until edges are lightly browned and leaves are crisp. Cool completely. Store in airtight container.

*MAKES 6 SERVINGS*

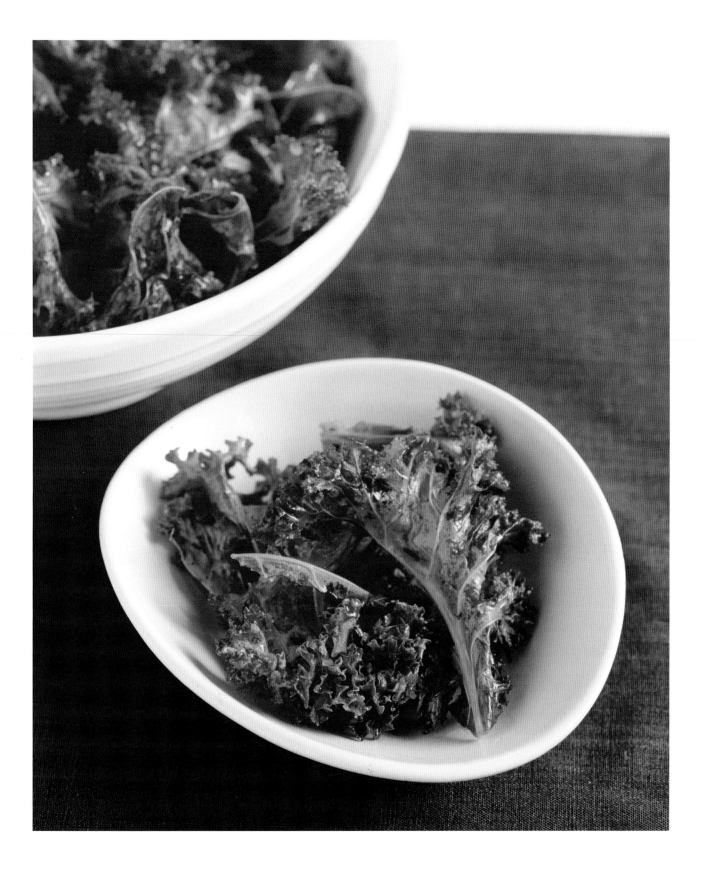

# Banana Bowties

1 cup peeled chopped ripe
  banana (about 2 medium)

¼ cup finely chopped walnuts
  or pecans

1 tablespoon packed brown
  sugar

20 square wonton wrappers

1 egg, beaten

  Chocolate syrup

1. Preheat air fryer to 370°F. Combine banana, nuts and brown sugar in small bowl; gently mix.

2. Arrange wonton wrappers, one at a time, on clean surface. Brush edges with egg. Place teaspoonful of banana filling in center. Fold wrapper in half, pressing edges to seal. Pinch center to form bowtie. Cover with plastic wrap and refrigerate until ready to cook.

3. Cook in small batches 8 to 10 minutes or until golden brown. Drizzle with chocolate syrup. Serve immediately.

*MAKES 20 BOWTIES*

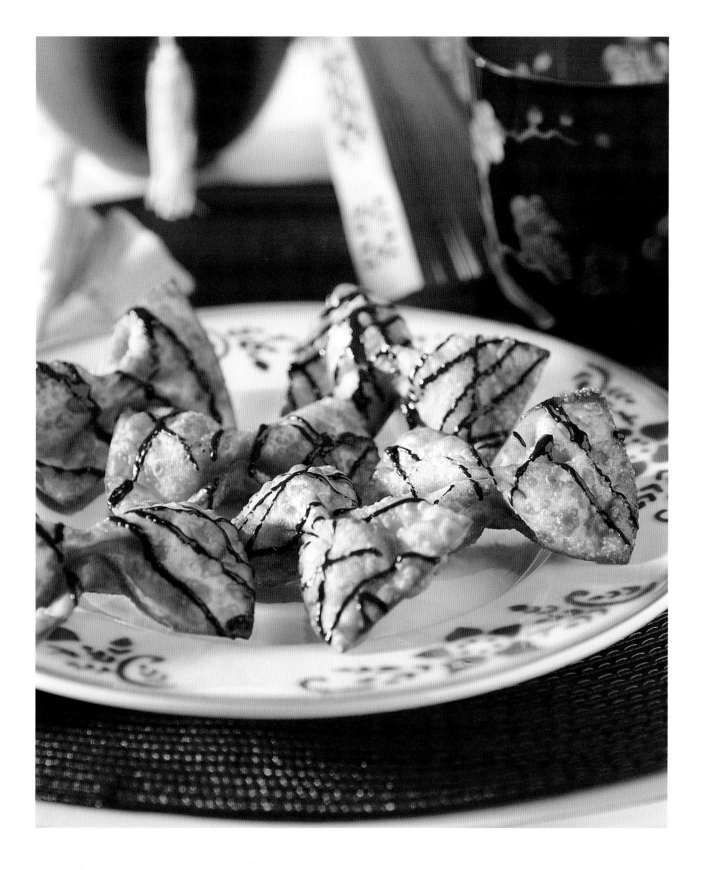

# Corn Tortilla Chips

6 (6-inch) corn tortillas,
  preferably day-old

½ teaspoon salt

Prepared guacamole

1. If tortillas are fresh, let stand, uncovered, in single layer on wire rack 1 to 2 hours to dry slightly.

2. Stack tortillas; cut tortillas into 6 or 8 equal wedges. Spray tortillas generously with nonstick olive oil cooking spray.

3. Preheat air fryer to 370°F.

4. Cook in batches 5 to 6 minutes, shaking halfway through cooking. Sprinkle chips with salt. Serve with guacamole.

*MAKES 6 DOZEN CHIPS*

Note: Tortilla chips are served with salsa as a snack, used as the base for nachos and used as scoops for guacamole, other dips or refried beans. They are best eaten fresh, but can be stored, tightly covered, in cool place 2 or 3 days.

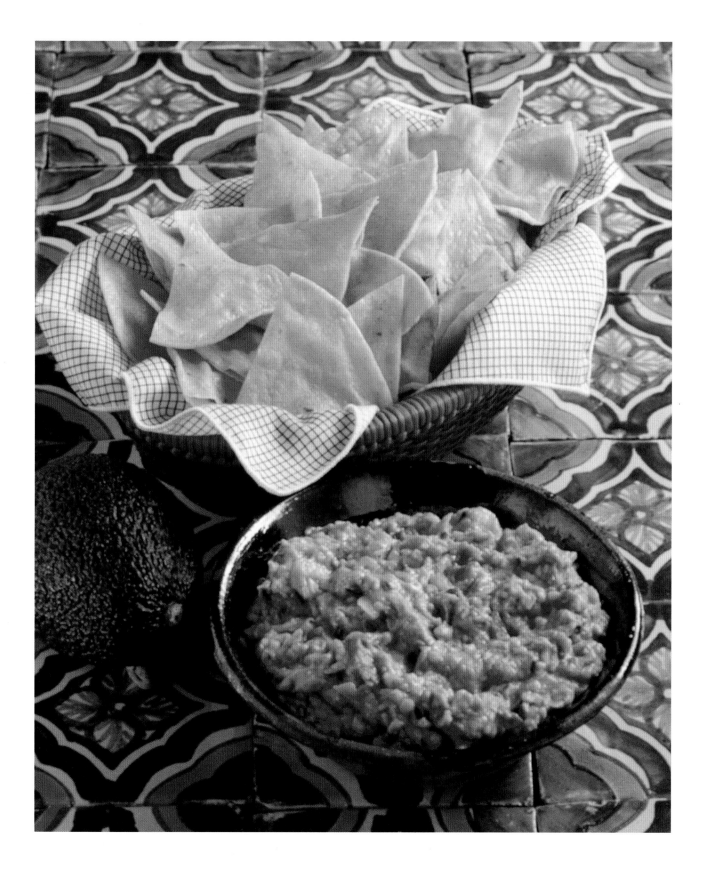

# Candied Nuts

1 egg white

1½ cups whole almonds

1½ cups pecan halves

1 cup powdered sugar

2 tablespoons lemon juice

2 teaspoons grated orange peel

1 teaspoon grated lemon peel

⅛ teaspoon ground nutmeg

1. Preheat air fryer to 300°F. Spray air fryer basket with nonstick cooking spray.

2. Beat egg white in medium bowl. Add almonds and pecans; stir until well coated. Combine powdered sugar, lemon juice, orange peel, lemon peel and nutmeg in medium bowl until evenly coated. Combine nuts and sugar mixture; toss until well coated.

3. Cook 20 to 22 minutes, shaking several times during cooking. Cool slightly. Store in airtight container up to 2 weeks.

*MAKES ABOUT 3 CUPS*

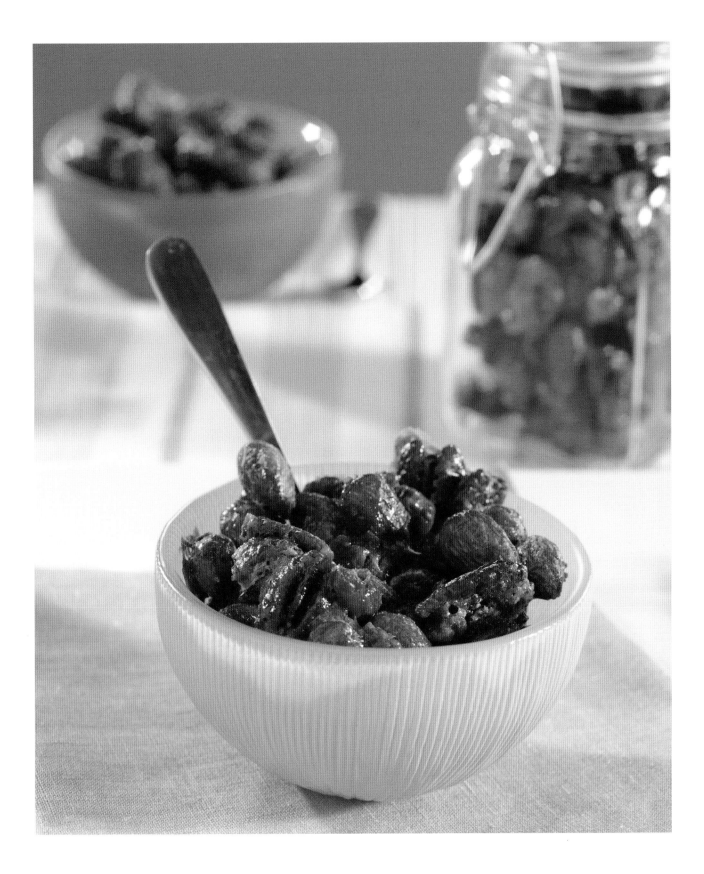

# Herbed Potato Chips

2 tablespoons minced fresh
  dill, thyme or rosemary
  leaves *or* 2 teaspoons
  dried dill weed, thyme
  or rosemary

¼ teaspoon garlic salt

⅛ teaspoon black pepper

2 unpeeled medium red
  potatoes (about ½ pound)

1¼ cups sour cream

1. Preheat air fryer to 390°F. Line air fryer basket with parchment paper; spray with nonstick cooking spray. Combine dill, garlic salt and pepper in small bowl; set aside.

2. Cut potatoes crosswise into very thin slices, about ¹⁄₁₆ inch thick. Pat dry with paper towels. Spray potatoes with cooking spray.

3. Cook in batches 8 to 10 minutes; shake. Spray with cooking spray; sprinkle evenly with seasoning mixture.

4. Cook 5 to 6 minutes or until golden brown. Cool. Serve with sour cream.

*MAKES 6 SERVINGS*

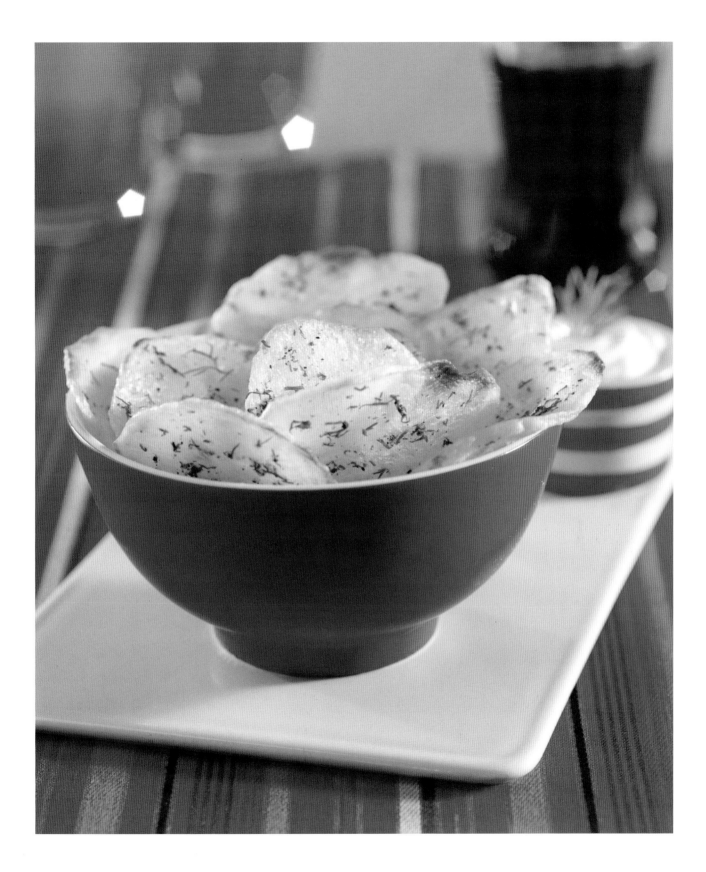

# Happy Apple Salsa with Baked Cinnamon Pita Chips

2 teaspoons sugar

¼ teaspoon ground cinnamon

2 pita bread rounds, split

1 tablespoon jelly or jam

1 medium apple, diced

1 tablespoon finely diced celery

1 tablespoon finely diced carrot

1 tablespoon golden raisins

1 teaspoon lemon juice

1. Preheat air fryer to 330°F.

2. Combine sugar and cinnamon in small bowl. Cut pita rounds into wedges. Spray with nonstick cooking spray; sprinkle with cinnamon-sugar.

3. Cook 8 to 10 minutes or until lightly browned. Set aside to cool.

4. Meanwhile, place jelly in medium microwavable bowl; microwave on HIGH 10 seconds. Stir in apple, celery, carrot, raisins and lemon juice. Serve salsa with pita chips.

*MAKES 3 SERVINGS*

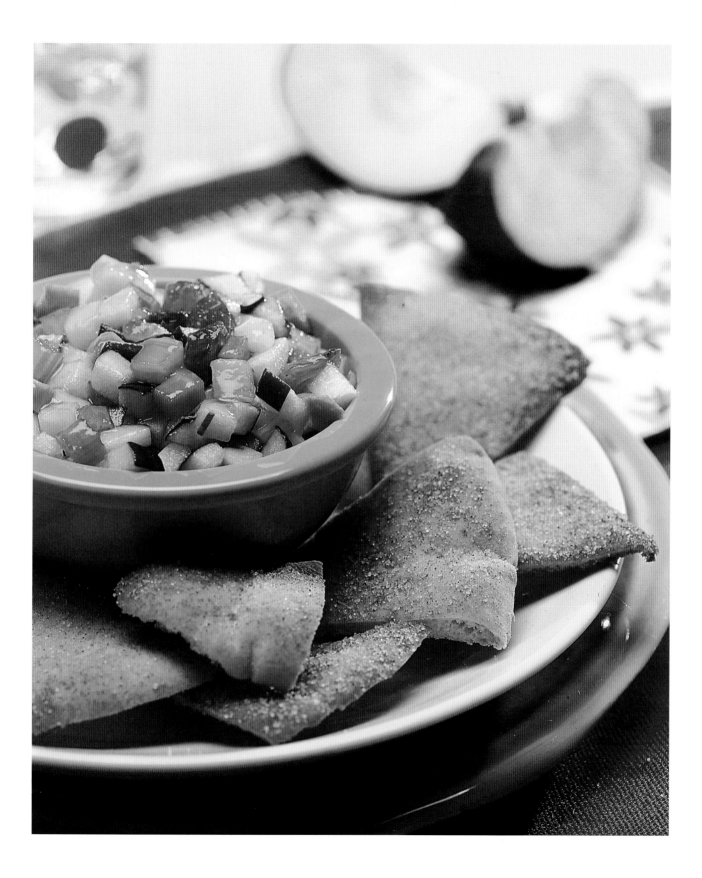

# Easy Wonton Chips

1 tablespoon soy sauce

2 teaspoons peanut or vegetable oil

½ teaspoon sugar

¼ teaspoon garlic salt

12 wonton wrappers

1. Preheat air fryer to 360°F. Combine soy sauce, oil, sugar and garlic salt in small bowl; mix well.

2. Cut each wonton wrapper diagonally in half. Spray with nonstick cooking spray. Brush soy sauce mixture lightly over both sides of wrappers.

3. Cook in batches 3 to 5 minutes or until crisp and lightly browned, turning halfway during cooking. Transfer to wire rack; cool completely.

*MAKES 2 DOZEN CHIPS*

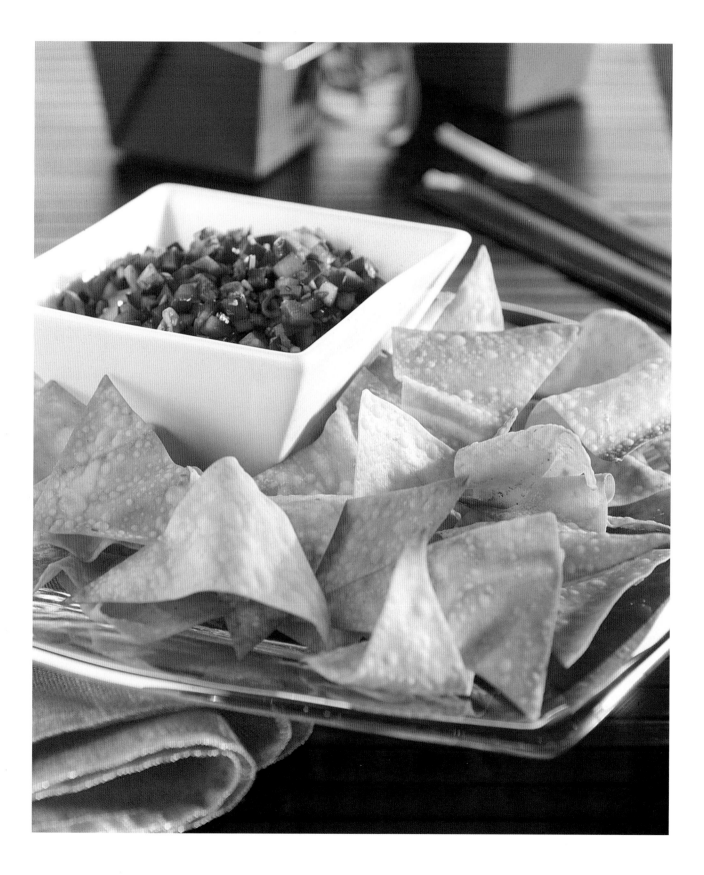

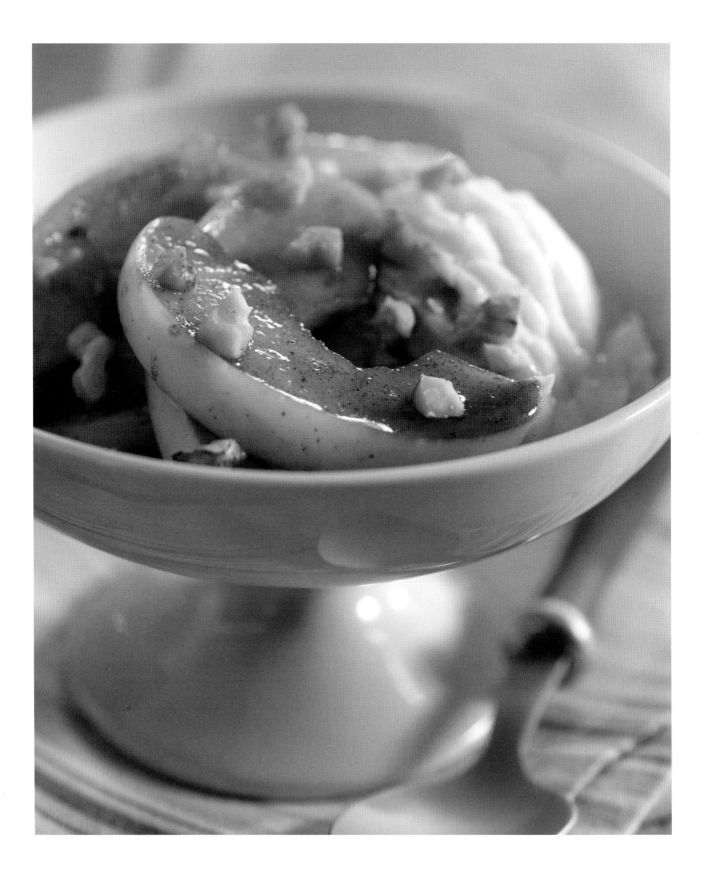

# Desserts

# Cherry Turnovers

1 can (21 ounces) cherry pie filling

2 teaspoons grated orange peel

1 package (15 ounces) refrigerated pie crusts (2 crusts)

All-purpose flour

1 egg yolk

1 tablespoon milk

1 tablespoon sugar

½ teaspoon ground cinnamon

1. Combine pie filling and orange peel in medium bowl.

2. Roll out one pie crust into 12-inch circle on lightly floured surface. Cut out six 4-inch circles with cookie cutter. Repeat with second crust.

3. Beat egg yolk and milk in small bowl until blended. Combine sugar and cinnamon in separate small bowl.

4. Spoon scant tablespoon pie filling mixture in center of each pastry circle. Brush edges of circles with egg yolk mixture; fold in half to enclose filling. Press edges together with fork to seal.

5. Cut slits in tops of turnovers with paring knife. Brush with remaining egg yolk mixture; sprinkle with cinnamon-sugar.

6. Preheat air fryer to 350°F. Cook 12 to 15 minutes or until golden brown. Remove to wire rack; cool slightly. Serve warm.

*MAKES 12 TURNOVERS*

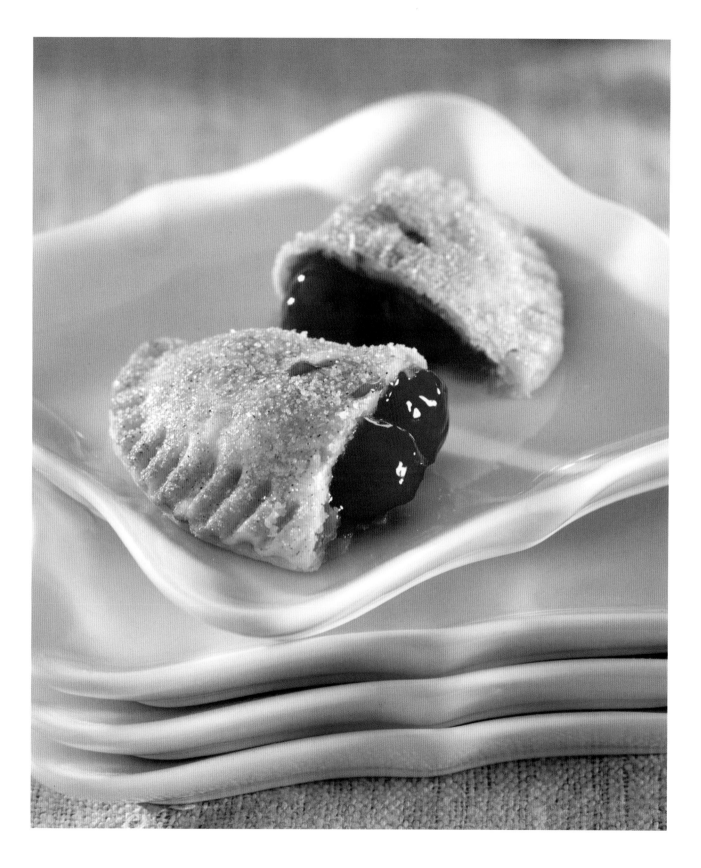

# Chocolate-Peanut Butter Bananas

¼ cup chocolate syrup

1 tablespoon peanut butter

1 large firm banana,
   unpeeled

1 teaspoon melted butter

1 tablespoon packed brown
   sugar

1 cup vanilla ice cream

2 tablespoons chopped
   peanuts

1. Place chocolate syrup in small microwavable bowl. Heat on HIGH in microwave 10 to 15 seconds until warm. Slowly whisk in peanut butter until well blended. Keep warm until ready to serve.

2. Preheat air fryer to 350°F. Line air fryer basket with foil or parchment paper. Cut unpeeled banana in half lengthwise. Brush cut sides with butter; place cut side down in air fryer basket. Cook 1½ to 2 minutes. Turn banana; spread brown sugar over banana. Cook 1 to 2 minutes or until brown sugar melts and banana softens.

3. Peel banana; cut each piece in half. Place two pieces in each serving dish. Top with ice cream. Drizzle with warm chocolate sauce; sprinkle with peanuts.

*MAKES 2 SERVINGS*

Note: To chop peanuts, place in small resealable food storage bag and crush slightly with a meat mallet.

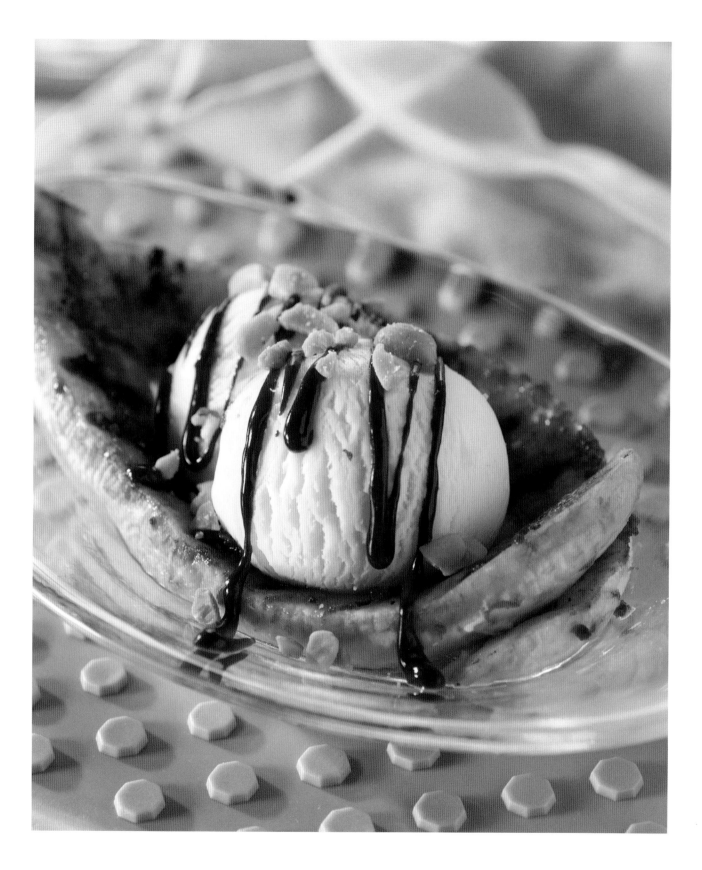

# Pineapple with Spiced Vanilla Sauce

3 ounces cream cheese

¼ cup granulated sugar

¼ cup half-and-half

¼ teaspoon pumpkin pie spice

¼ teaspoon vanilla

1 sheet (14×12 inches) heavy-duty foil

2 teaspoons butter

2 thick round slices fresh pineapple, skin and eyes trimmed

1 tablespoon light brown sugar

1. Place cream cheese, granulated sugar, half-and-half, pumpkin pie spice and vanilla in food processor or blender; process until smooth. Refrigerate.

2. Coat center of foil sheet with butter. Place pineapple slices side by side on foil. Sprinkle with brown sugar. Fold up sides and ends of foil around pineapple, leaving top open. Place in air fryer basket.

3. Preheat air fryer to 350°F. Cook 10 to 12 minutes or until surface of pineapple is bubbling and browned.

4. Transfer pineapple to serving plates. Serve immediately with cream cheese mixture.

*MAKES 2 SERVINGS*

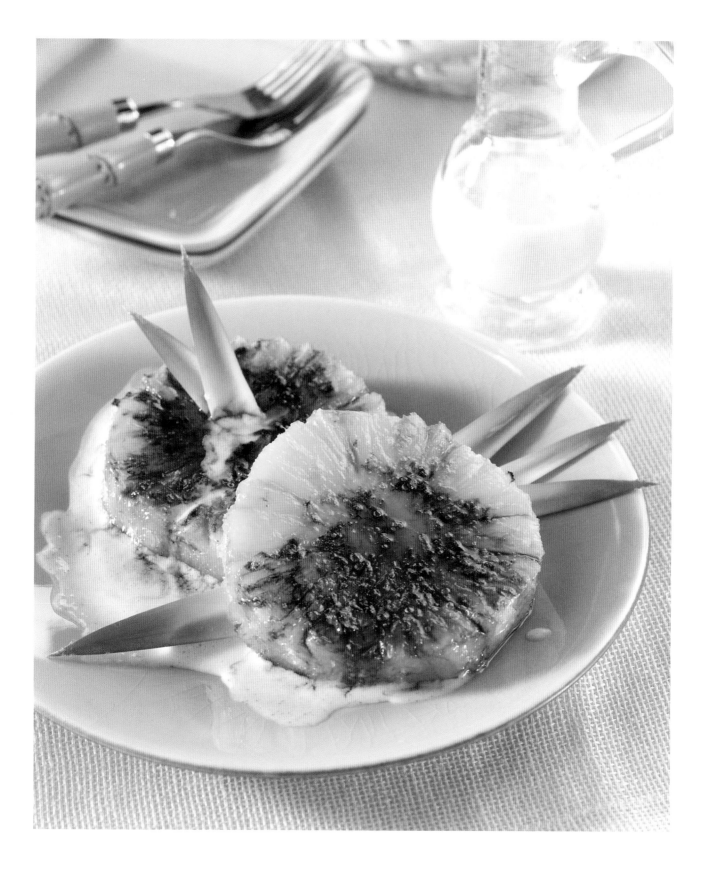

# Peaches
# with Raspberry Sauce

1 package (10 ounces) frozen raspberries, thawed

1½ teaspoons lemon juice

2 tablespoons packed brown sugar

½ teaspoon ground cinnamon

1 can (15 ounces) peach halves in juice (4 halves)

Foil

2 teaspoons butter

Fresh mint sprigs

1. Combine raspberries and lemon juice in food processor fitted with metal blade; process until smooth. Refrigerate until ready to serve.

2. Preheat air fryer to 350°F.

3. Combine brown sugar and cinnamon in medium bowl; coat peach halves with mixture. Place peach halves, cut sides up, on foil. Dot with butter. Fold foil over peaches, leaving head space for steam; seal foil. Place packet in air fryer basket.

4. Cook 10 minutes or until peaches are soft and lightly browned.

5. To serve, spoon 2 tablespoons raspberry sauce over each peach half. Garnish with fresh mint sprig.

*MAKES 4 SERVINGS*

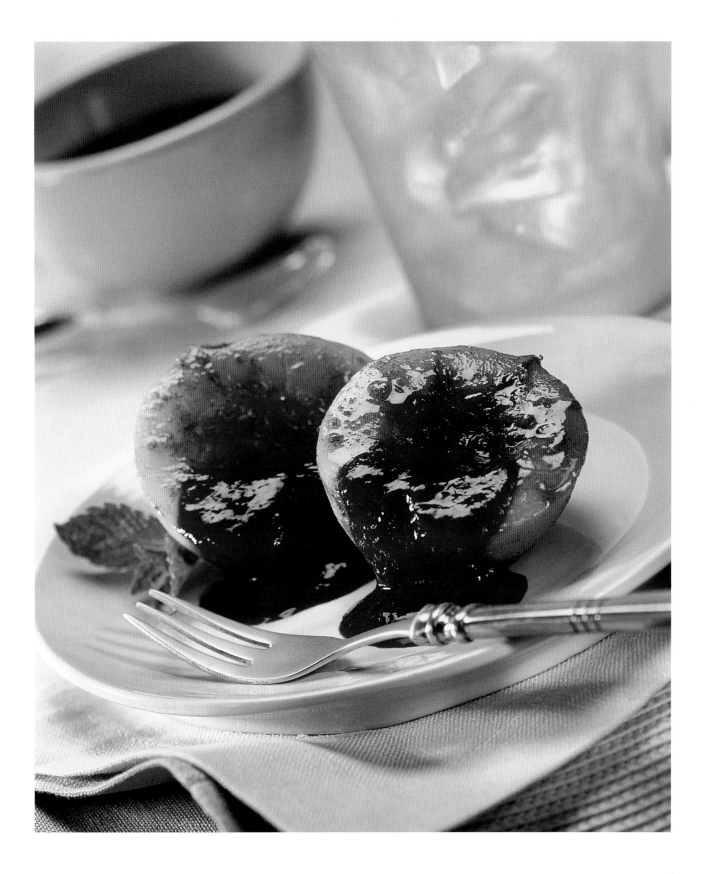

# Sautéed Apples Supreme

2 small Granny Smith apples
*or* 1 large Granny Smith
apple

1 teaspoon butter, melted

¼ cup unsweetened apple
juice or cider

1 teaspoon packed brown
sugar

½ teaspoon ground cinnamon

⅔ cup vanilla ice cream or
frozen yogurt (optional)

1 tablespoon chopped
walnuts, toasted

1. Preheat air fryer to 350°F. Spray air fryer basket with nonstick cooking spray.

2. Cut apples into quarters; remove cores and cut into ½-inch-thick slices. Toss butter and apples in medium bowl.

3. Combine apple juice, brown sugar and cinnamon in small bowl; pour over apples.

4. Cook 6 to 8 minutes or until soft and lightly golden, shaking halfway through cooking. Transfer to serving bowls; serve with ice cream, if desired. Sprinkle with walnuts.

*MAKES 2 SERVINGS*

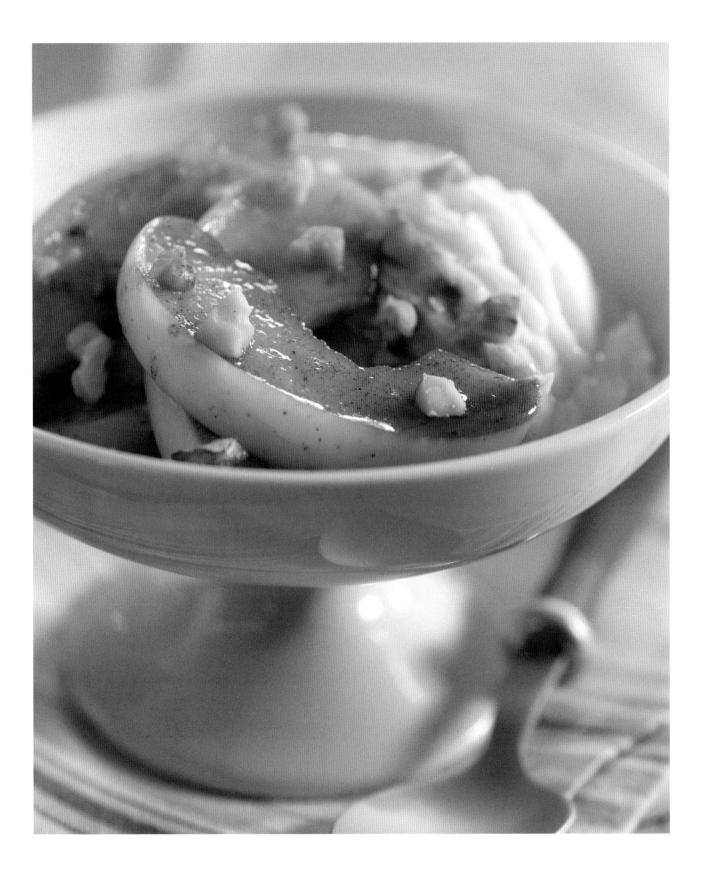

# Double-Berry Shortcakes

## STRAWBERRY FILLING

- 2 to 3 cups fresh sliced strawberries
- 1 tablespoon sugar

## RASPBERRY SAUCE

- 1 package (10 ounces) frozen unsweetened raspberries, thawed
- 1 tablespoon sugar

## SHORTCAKES

- 1 package (9 ounces) yellow cake mix without pudding in the mix
- 1 egg
- ½ cup cold water
- 2 teaspoons freshly grated lemon peel

## WHIPPED CREAM

- ½ cup whipping cream
- 1 tablespoon sugar

1. Combine 2 cups strawberries and 1 tablespoon sugar in medium bowl. Let stand, 30 minutes to 2 hours, stirring occasionally, until sugar dissolves.

2. Meanwhile, place raspberries in fine wire sieve over medium bowl. Press raspberries through sieve with rubber spatula. Discard seeds and solids. Add 1 tablespoon sugar; stir until sugar is dissolved. Set aside.

3. Preheat air fryer to 330°F. Spray eight 2½-inch silicone muffin cups with nonstick cooking spray.

4. Combine cake mix, egg and water in large bowl; beat according to package directions. Stir in lemon peel. Spoon batter evenly into prepared muffin cups.

5. Cook in batches 10 to 12 minutes or until toothpick inserted into centers comes out clean. Transfer to wire rack; cool completely.

6. Beat whipping cream and 1 tablespoon sugar in chilled medium bowl with electric mixer at high speed until soft peaks form.

7. Split shortcakes in half horizontally; place bottoms on eight plates. Spoon about ¼ cup strawberries on each cake; drizzle with 1 tablespoon raspberry sauce. Top with 2 tablespoons whipped cream. Cover with shortcake tops. Dollop evenly with remaining whipped cream; drizzle with remaining raspberry sauce. Refrigerate leftovers.

*MAKES 8 SERVINGS*

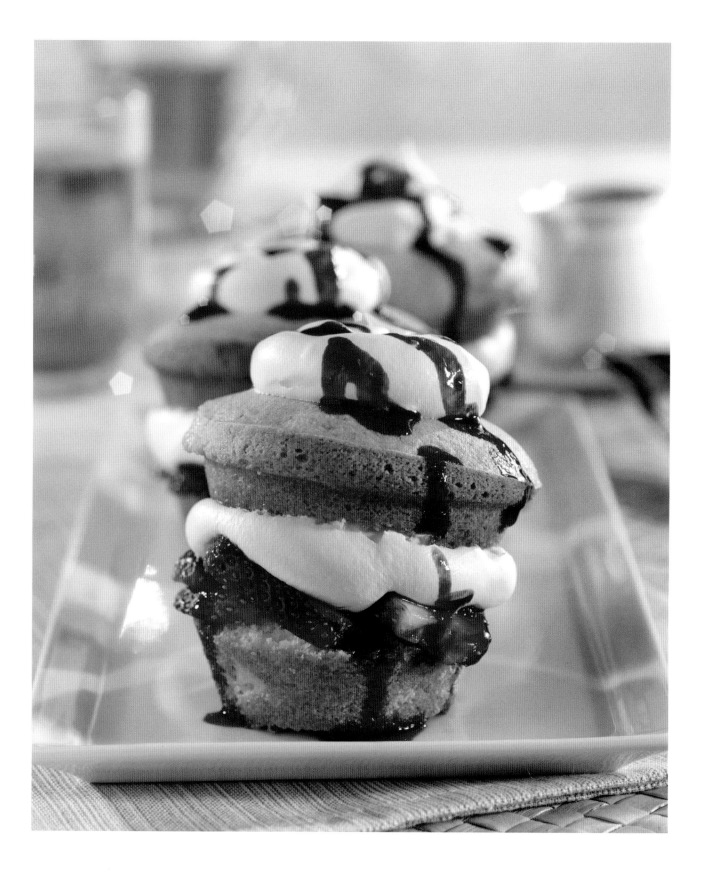

# Chocolate Cherry Turnovers

1 can (8 ounces) refrigerated crescent rolls

¾ cup semisweet chocolate chips, divided

½ cup canned cherry pie filling

1. Preheat air fryer to 360°F. Spray air fryer basket with nonstick cooking spray.

2. Unroll dough onto clean work surface; separate into 4 rectangles. Press perforations firmly to seal. Cut off corners of rectangles with sharp paring knife to form oval shapes.

3. Place 1 tablespoon chocolate chips on half of each oval; top with 2 tablespoons pie filling. Sprinkle with additional 1 tablespoon chocolate chips. Fold dough over filling; press edges to seal. Crimp edges with fork, if desired.

4. Cook in batches 8 to 10 minutes or until golden brown. Cool on wire rack 5 minutes. Melt remaining chocolate chips and drizzle over turnovers. Serve warm.

*MAKES 4 TURNOVERS*

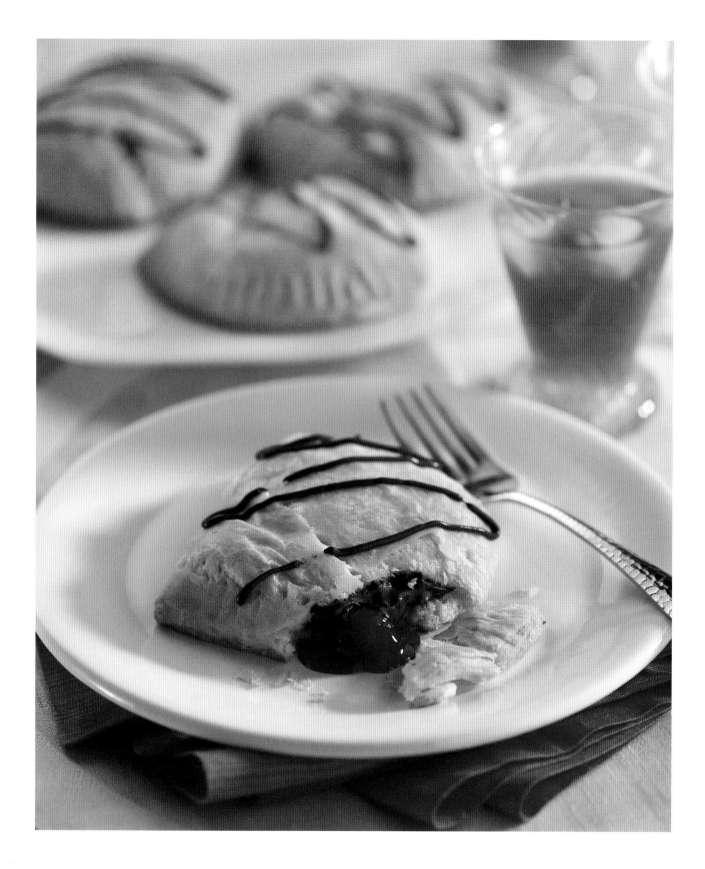

# Baked Cinnamon Apples

2  large Granny Smith apples

2  sheets heavy-duty foil,
   lightly sprayed with
   nonstick cooking spray

2  tablespoons packed brown
   sugar

2  tablespoons dried
   cranberries

½  teaspoon ground cinnamon

2  teaspoons butter

   Vanilla ice cream

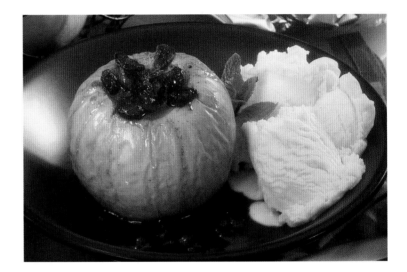

1. Preheat air fryer to 350°F. Core apples. Using paring knife, trim off ½-inch strip around top of each apple. Place each apple in center of foil sheet.

2. Mix brown sugar, cranberries and cinnamon in small bowl. Fill inside of apples with sugar mixture, sprinkling any excess around pared rim. Place butter on sugar mixture; press gently.

3. Double fold sides and ends of foil to seal packets, leaving head space for heat circulation. Place packets in air fryer basket.

4. Cook 12 to 14 minutes or until apple is slightly softened. Transfer apples to bowls; spoon remaining liquid over apples. Serve warm apples with ice cream.

*MAKES 2 SERVINGS*

# Index

# METRIC CONVERSION CHART

## VOLUME MEASUREMENTS (dry)

1/8 teaspoon = 0.5 mL
1/4 teaspoon = 1 mL
1/2 teaspoon = 2 mL
3/4 teaspoon = 4 mL
1 teaspoon = 5 mL
1 tablespoon = 15 mL
2 tablespoons = 30 mL
1/4 cup = 60 mL
1/3 cup = 75 mL
1/2 cup = 125 mL
2/3 cup = 150 mL
3/4 cup = 175 mL
1 cup = 250 mL
2 cups = 1 pint = 500 mL
3 cups = 750 mL
4 cups = 1 quart = 1 L

## VOLUME MEASUREMENTS (fluid)

1 fluid ounce (2 tablespoons) = 30 mL
4 fluid ounces (1/2 cup) = 125 mL
8 fluid ounces (1 cup) = 250 mL
12 fluid ounces (1 1/2 cups) = 375 mL
16 fluid ounces (2 cups) = 500 mL

## WEIGHTS (mass)

1/2 ounce = 15 g
1 ounce = 30 g
3 ounces = 90 g
4 ounces = 120 g
8 ounces = 225 g
10 ounces = 285 g
12 ounces = 360 g
16 ounces = 1 pound = 450 g

## DIMENSIONS

1/16 inch = 2 mm
1/8 inch = 3 mm
1/4 inch = 6 mm
1/2 inch = 1.5 cm
3/4 inch = 2 cm
1 inch = 2.5 cm

## OVEN TEMPERATURES

250°F = 120°C
275°F = 140°C
300°F = 150°C
325°F = 160°C
350°F = 180°C
375°F = 190°C
400°F = 200°C
425°F = 220°C
450°F = 230°C

## BAKING PAN SIZES

| Utensil | Size in Inches/Quarts | Metric Volume | Size in Centimeters |
|---|---|---|---|
| Baking or Cake Pan (square or rectangular) | 8×8×2 | 2 L | 20×20×5 |
| | 9×9×2 | 2.5 L | 23×23×5 |
| | 12×8×2 | 3 L | 30×20×5 |
| | 13×9×2 | 3.5 L | 33×23×5 |
| Loaf Pan | 8×4×3 | 1.5 L | 20×10×7 |
| | 9×5×3 | 2 L | 23×13×7 |
| Round Layer Cake Pan | 8×1½ | 1.2 L | 20×4 |
| | 9×1½ | 1.5 L | 23×4 |
| Pie Plate | 8×1¼ | 750 mL | 20×3 |
| | 9×1¼ | 1 L | 23×3 |
| Baking Dish or Casserole | 1 quart | 1 L | — |
| | 1½ quart | 1.5 L | — |
| | 2 quart | 2 L | — |